Atlas of Cardiac Surgery

Atlas of Cardiac Surgery

William A. Baumgartner, MD
Cardiac Surgeon-in-Charge, Professor of Surgery,
Division of Cardiac Surgery, The Johns Hopkins Hospital
Baltimore, Maryland

R. Scott Stuart, MD
Associate Professor of Surgery, Division of Cardiac Surgery
The Johns Hopkins Hospital, Baltimore, Maryland

Vincent L. Gott, MD
Professor Emeritus of Surgery
The Johns Hopkins University School of Medicine
Co-Director
The Dana and Albert "Cubby" Broccoli Center for Aortic Diseases
The Johns Hopkins Hospital, Baltimore, Maryland

Leon Schlossberg
Department of Art as Applied to Medicine
The Johns Hopkins Hospital, Baltimore, Maryland
(Deceased)

HANLEY & BELFUS, INC. / Philadelphia

Publisher: HANLEY & BELFUS, INC.
              Medical Publishers
              210 South 13th Street
              Philadelphia, PA 19107
              (215) 546-7293; 800-962-1892
              FAX (215) 790-9330
              Web site: http://www.hanleyandbelfus.com

Note to the reader: Although the information in this book has been carefully reviewed for correctness of dosage and indications, neither the authors nor the editor nor the publisher can accept any legal responsibility for any errors or omissions that may be made. Neither the publisher nor the editor makes any warranty, expressed or implied, with respect to the material contained herein. Before prescribing any drug, the reader must review the manufacturer's current product information (package inserts) for accepted indications, absolute dosage recommendations, and other information pertinent to the safe and effective use of the product described.

Library of Congress Cataloging-in-Publication Data

Atlas of cardiac surgery / edited by William A. Baumgartner . . . [et al.]
        p. ; cm.
      Includes index.
      ISBN 1-56053-310-2 (alk. paper)
        1. Heart—Surgery—Atlases. I. Baumgartner, William A.
      [DNLM: 1. Thoracic Surgical Procedures—Atlases. 2. Cardiovascular Surgical
Procedures— Atlases.   WG 17 A8815 2000]
      RD598.A926 2000
      617.4'12'00222—dc21
                                                                   99-052486

ATLAS OF CARDIAC SURGERY   ISBN 1-56053-310-2

Last digit is the print number: 9 8 7 6 5 4 3 2 1

Contents

Contributors

Duke E. Cameron, MD
Associate Professor, Department of Surgery, The Johns Hopkins Hospital, Johns Hopkins University School of Medicine, Baltimore, Maryland

John V. Conte, MD
Assistant Professor, Department of Surgery, Director of Heart and Heart-Lung Transplantation, Co-Director of Lung Transplantation, Johns Hopkins University School of Medicine, Baltimore, Maryland

James L. Cox, MD
Professor and Chairman, Cardiovascular and Thoracic Surgery; Surgical Director, Georgetown University Cardiovascular Research Institute, Georgetown University Medical Center, Washington, D.C.

J. Mark Redmond, MD
Assistant Professor, Department of Surgery; Co-Director, The Dana and Albert "Cubby" Broccoli Center for Aortic Diseases, The Johns Hopkins University School of Medicine, Baltimore, Maryland

G. Melville Williams, MD
Professor, Department of Surgery, The Johns Hopkins University School of Medicine, Baltimore, Maryland

Leon Schlossberg, 1912–1999

On November 29, 1944, the era of modern cardiac surgery was ushered in at the Johns Hopkins Hospital when Dr. Alfred Blalock performed a subclavian artery–pulmonary artery shunt operation on a child with tetralogy of Fallot. How fortuitous it was that, a few months later, a young medical illustrator, Leon Schlossberg, returned from World War II naval service to join the Department of Art as Applied to Medicine at Johns Hopkins. Dr. Blalock recognized Mr. Schlossberg's exceptional illustrative talents and arranged for him to be the primary illustrator for all cardiac surgical publications emanating from this institution.

Fortunately, for those of us here at Johns Hopkins, Leon Schlossberg continued as our principal medical illustrator right up until a few months before he passed away on December 19, 1999.

Leon Schlossberg's illustrative talents were first recognized by Max Brödel, the father of modern medical illustration. Brödel had come to Johns Hopkins in 1911 to establish the Department of Art as Applied to Medicine. Leon met Max Brödel in the early 1930s when he was a student at the Maryland Institute of Art. Brödel invited Leon to be a student in his department, and on graduation he remained as an instructor. Brödel had developed a remarkable new illustrative method known as the "Brödel half-tone" technique; it was his student, Leon Schlossberg, who brought this technique to its ultimate artistic quality over the past six decades. Leon's notes on this technique are included in these opening pages.

Those of us who have collaborated on this atlas deeply appreciate the opportunity that we have had to work with one of the preeminent medical illustrators of this past century.

Vincent L. Gott, M.D.

A Note on the Art Materials
and Techniques
Used in this Book

Max Brödel, the world-famous medical illustrator, was teacher of medical illustration at Johns Hopkins Medical School from 1910 to 1940. He realized early in his career that there was no existing drawing board that would satisfactorily represent the characteristics of human tissue: the textures, translucency, highlights, shadows, and other characteristics evident at surgical operations. Characteristics applied by white pigment looked very artificial. Brödel contacted a paper manufacturer and worked with them to develop a calcium-coated board, or "stipple board," which indeed proved to be "custom made" for creating high-quality medical illustrations.

The technique for using the board begins with the creation of a sketch of the subject matter using a soft carbon pencil. The sketch is then rubbed onto another blank sheet using a blunt metallic instrument, resulting in a negative impression; this, in turn, is attached to the calcium board and rubbed onto the surface, resulting in a faint positive. The details from the original sketch are then drawn in. A soft bristle brush is rubbed over the entire drawing to blend the details. Shading is accomplished by brushing on dust from a carbon pencil. Soft highlights are achieved using a soft rubber eraser, bringing out the natural calcium highlights. Brilliant highlights and light-reflective surfaces are produced by scratching with a scalpel blade. Black accents and rich black tones are readily applied with pencil, and shadows are produced with flat sable brushes.

This same technique invented by Brödel has been used in the creation of the drawings in the *Atlas of Cardiac Surgery*.

Leon Schlossberg

Preface

This *Atlas of Cardiac Surgery* is primarily designed as a working atlas to aid residents, fellows, and attendings in cardiac surgery. Its focus is on procedures which apply to adults, although the chapters on transplantation are appropriate for patients of all ages. Details of the procedures reflect the philosophy and practice of the surgical group at Johns Hopkins. We do not feel that the methods described here denote the only or best way of performing an operation. All operations continue to evolve technically. This is especially true in the chapters pertaining to minimally invasive techniques. There are many pathways to a good outcome. We have tried to add notations on certain pearls or pitfalls which apply to the given operation.

Why another atlas on cardiac surgery? This atlas illustrates the techniques of operations which have worked well for our practice and provides the one thing that previous atlases lack: the wonderful illustrations by Mr. Leon Schlossberg. Mr. Schlossberg graced the halls of Johns Hopkins for longer than any of the authors of this atlas, and his contributions to the field of surgery and medical illustration are truly legendary. It was the chance to work with Leon which drew our faculty to this book and it has been an honor, privilege, and delight to have worked closely with him. Sadly, this book has proved to be Leon's last full work, as he passed away in December of 1999. He is sorely missed as a colleague and as a friend. We hope the reader will agree that this atlas reflects the fine art of which Leon was a master. Our thanks and our hearts are with him always.

Finally, the expert guidance, help, and patience of Mr. William Lamsback and his staff at Hanley & Belfus Medical Publishers are greatly appreciated. Their skills, editing, and layout have placed Mr. Schlossberg's art within an excellent frame.

William A. Baumgartner, MD
R. Scott Stuart, MD
Vincent L. Gott, MD

Chapter 1

Cardiothoracic Anatomy
An Atlas

Anterior View of the Heart

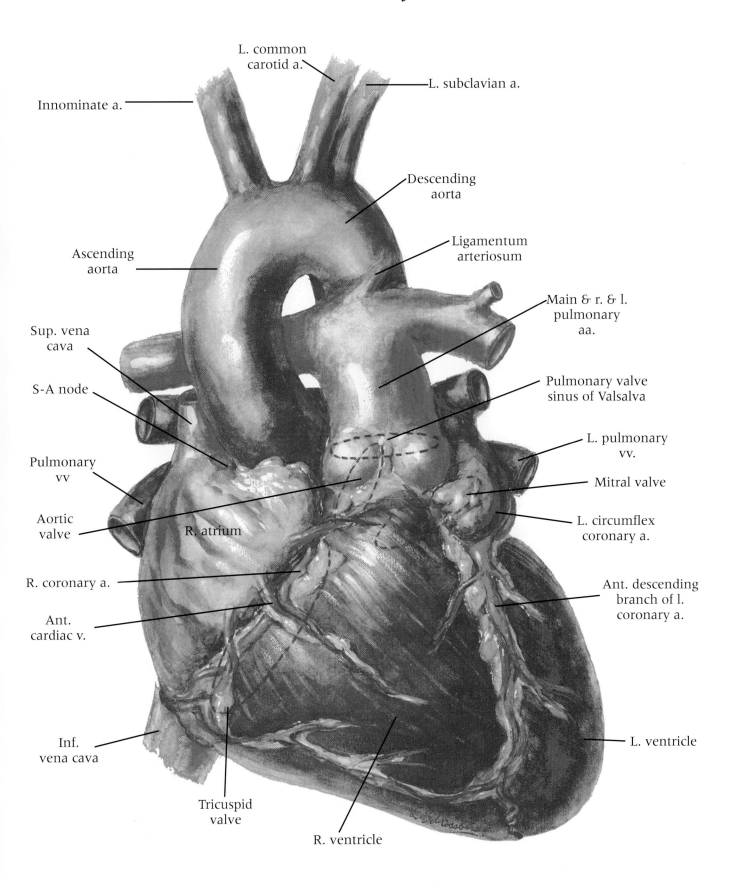

L. common
carotid a.

L. subclavian a.

Innominate a.

Descending
aorta

Ligamentum
arteriosum

Ascending
aorta

Main & r. & l.
pulmonary
aa.

Sup. vena
cava

Pulmonary valve
sinus of Valsalva

S-A node

L. pulmonary
vv.

Pulmonary
vv

Mitral valve

Aortic
valve

R. atrium

L. circumflex
coronary a.

R. coronary a.

Ant. descending
branch of l.
coronary a.

Ant.
cardiac v.

Inf.
vena cava

L. ventricle

Tricuspid
valve

R. ventricle

Three-Chamber View of the Heart

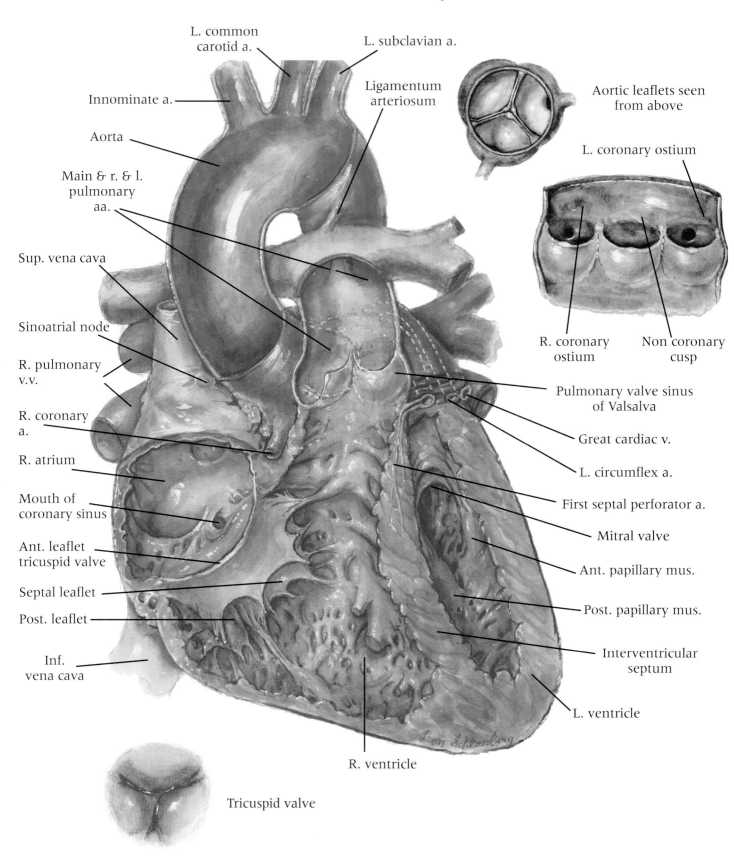

L. common carotid a.

L. subclavian a.

Ligamentum arteriosum

Innominate a.

Aorta

Main & r. & l. pulmonary aa.

Sup. vena cava

Sinoatrial node

R. pulmonary v.v.

R. coronary a.

R. atrium

Mouth of coronary sinus

Ant. leaflet tricuspid valve

Septal leaflet

Post. leaflet

Inf. vena cava

Aortic leaflets seen from above

L. coronary ostium

R. coronary ostium

Non coronary cusp

Pulmonary valve sinus of Valsalva

Great cardiac v.

L. circumflex a.

First septal perforator a.

Mitral valve

Ant. papillary mus.

Post. papillary mus.

Interventricular septum

L. ventricle

R. ventricle

Tricuspid valve

Innervation of the Heart

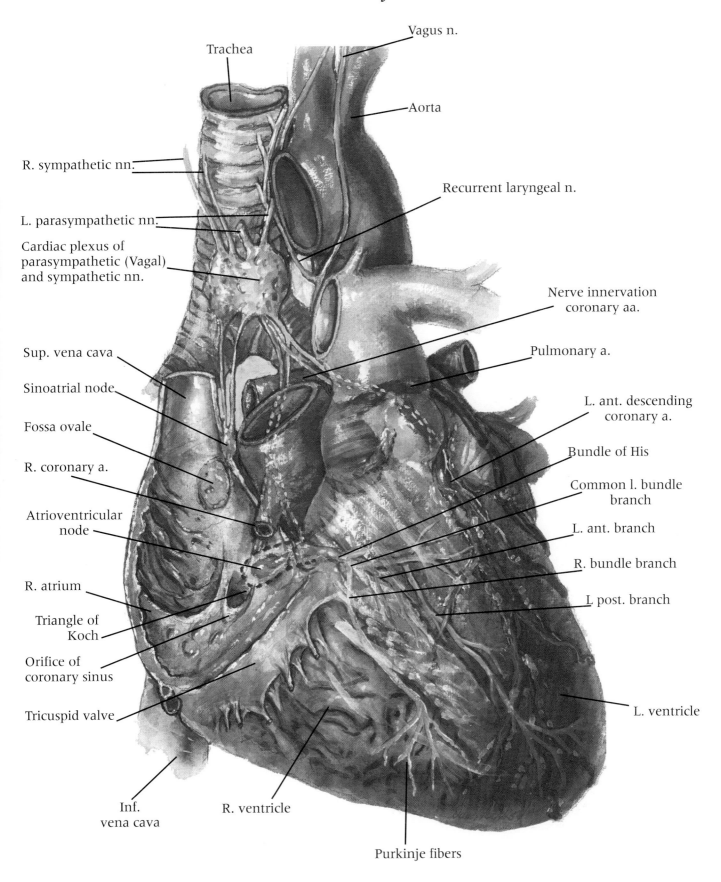

Trachea

Vagus n.

Aorta

R. sympathetic nn.

Recurrent laryngeal n.

L. parasympathetic nn.

Cardiac plexus of
parasympathetic (Vagal)
and sympathetic nn.

Nerve innervation
coronary aa.

Sup. vena cava

Pulmonary a.

Sinoatrial node

L. ant. descending
coronary a.

Fossa ovale

Bundle of His

R. coronary a.

Common l. bundle
branch

Atrioventricular
node

L. ant. branch

R. bundle branch

R. atrium

L post. branch

Triangle of
Koch

Orifice of
coronary sinus

L. ventricle

Tricuspid valve

Inf.
vena cava

R. ventricle

Purkinje fibers

Posterior View of the Heart

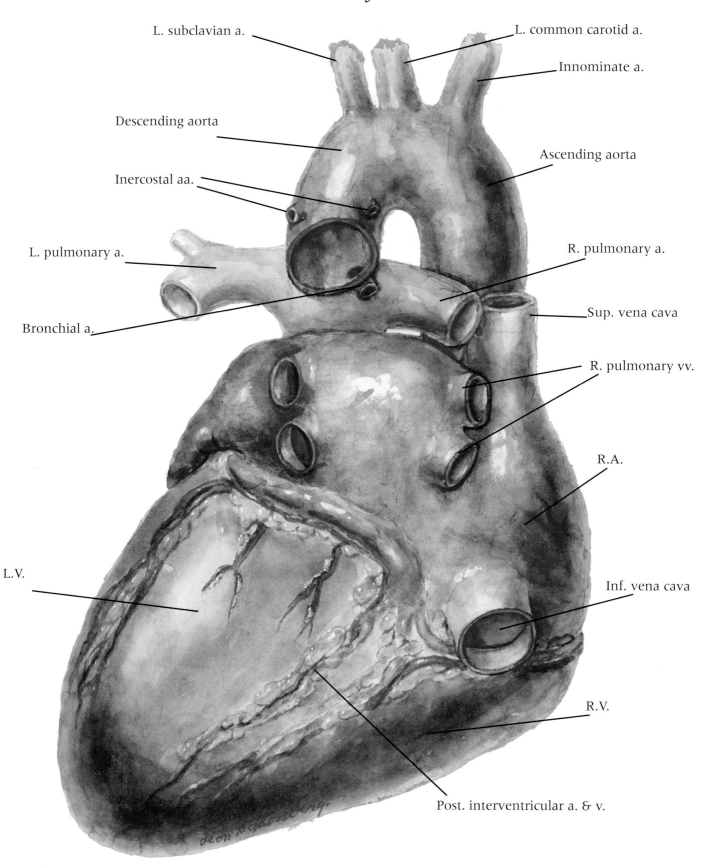

L. subclavian a.

L. common carotid a.

Innominate a.

Descending aorta

Inercostal aa.

Ascending aorta

L. pulmonary a.

R. pulmonary a.

Bronchial a.

Sup. vena cava

R. pulmonary vv.

R.A.

L.V.

Inf. vena cava

R.V.

Post. interventricular a. & v.

Pericardium

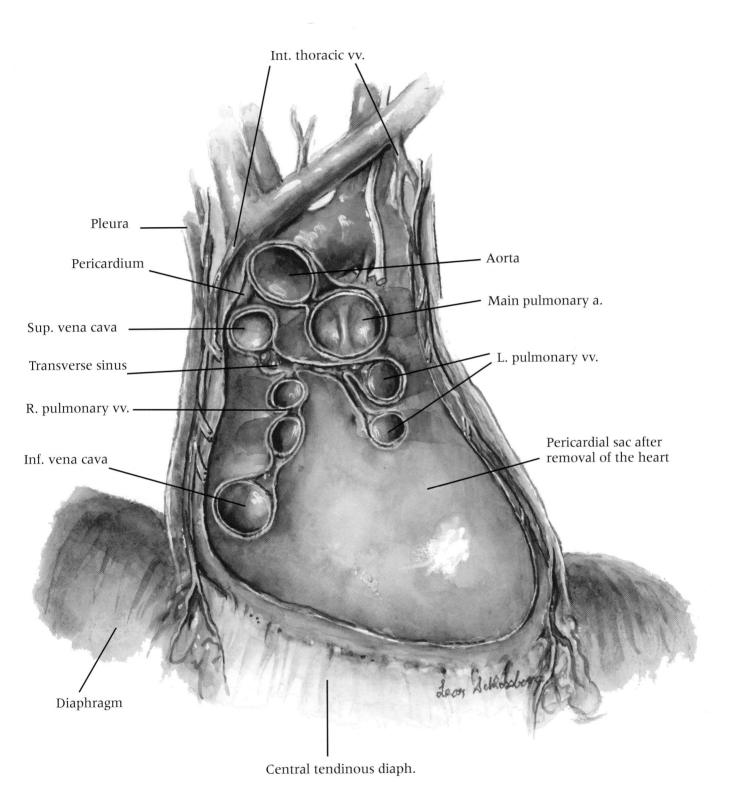

Int. thoracic vv.

Pleura

Pericardium

Sup. vena cava

Transverse sinus

R. pulmonary vv.

Inf. vena cava

Diaphragm

Central tendinous diaph.

Aorta

Main pulmonary a.

L. pulmonary vv.

Pericardial sac after removal of the heart

Arterial Anatomy of the Chest

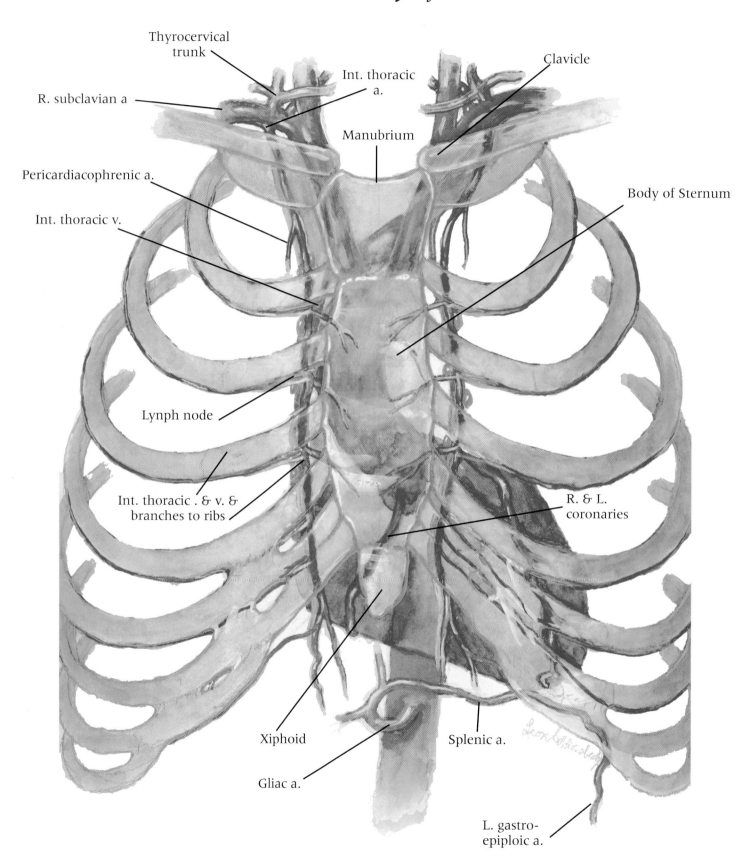

Thyrocervical trunk

Int. thoracic a.

Clavicle

R. subclavian a

Manubrium

Pericardiacophrenic a.

Body of Sternum

Int. thoracic v.

Lynph node

Int. thoracic . & v. & branches to ribs

R. & L. coronaries

Xiphoid

Splenic a.

Gliac a.

L. gastro-epiploic a.

Right Side of the Mediastinum

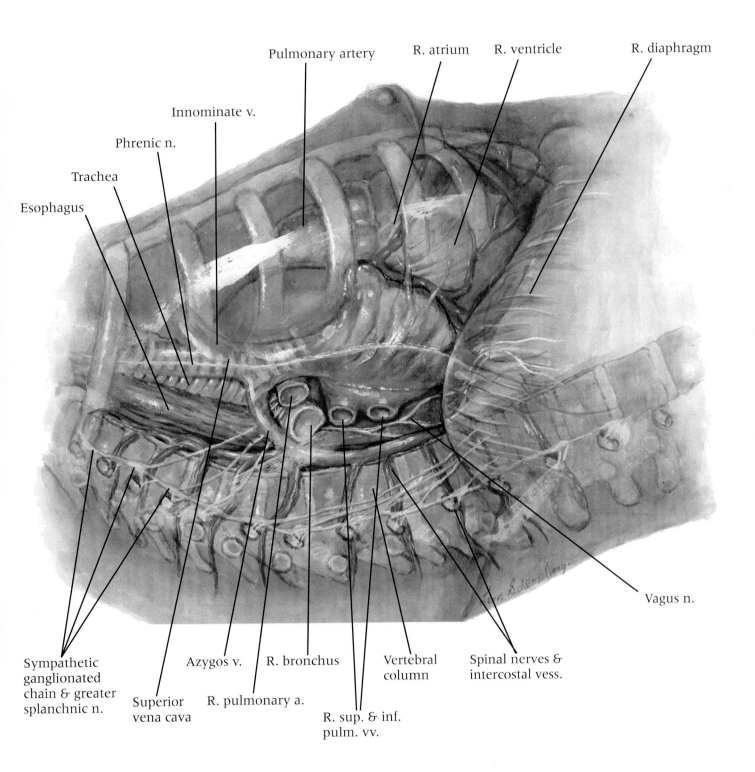

Pulmonary artery

R. atrium

R. ventricle

R. diaphragm

Innominate v.

Phrenic n.

Trachea

Esophagus

Vagus n.

Sympathetic
ganglionated
chain & greater
splanchnic n.

Azygos v.

R. bronchus

Vertebral
column

Spinal nerves &
intercostal vess.

Superior
vena cava

R. pulmonary a.

R. sup. & inf.
pulm. vv.

Left Side of the Mediastinum

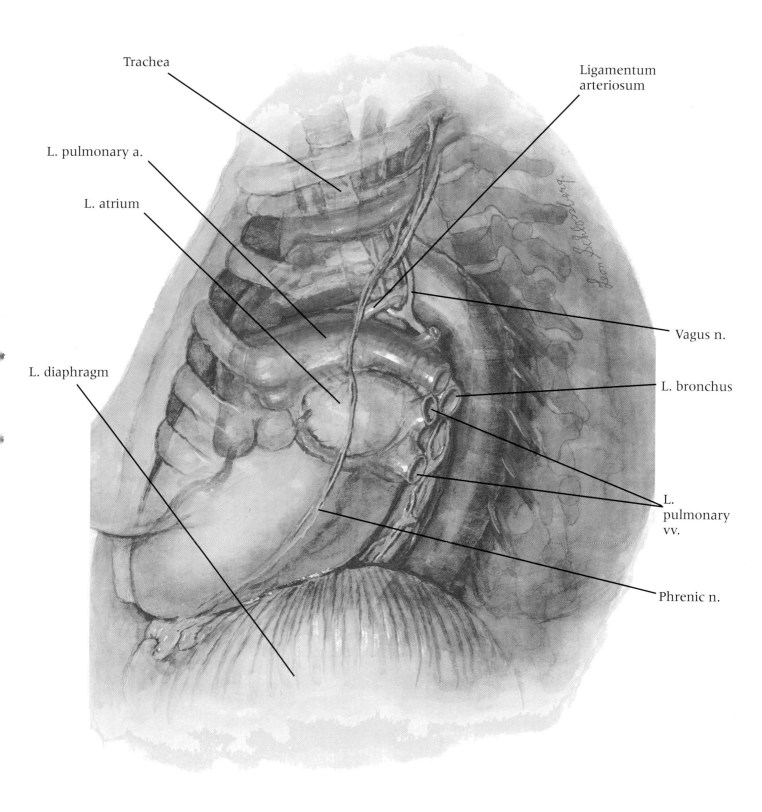

Trachea

Ligamentum arteriosum

L. pulmonary a.

L. atrium

Vagus n.

L. diaphragm

L. bronchus

L. pulmonary vv.

Phrenic n.

Chapter 2

Coronary Artery Bypass Grafting

John V. Conte, M.D.

Introduction

Coronary artery bypass grafting is the most commonly performed operation in cardiac surgery. The operation is performed through a standard midline sternotomy incision. The incision extends from the sternal notch to the xiphoid. The sternum is divided with an oscillating sternal saw. An internal mammary artery retractor is placed, and the left internal mammary artery is harvested from the undersurface of the left hemithorax. It is filled with a solution of dilute papaverine and wrapped in a sponge soaked in the same papaverine solution. It is then placed in the left upper mediastinum, out of the way, to be used later in the operation. The mammary retractor is removed and a standard retractor is placed. The sternum is widely separated. The pericardium is opened wide and the cut ends are sutured to the retractor to expose the heart and lift it up into the operative field. The patient is then systemically heparinized and then cannulated for cardiopulmonary bypass. A single arterial perfusion catheter and a dual-stage venous cannula are placed in the distal ascending aorta and right atrium through purse-string sutures secured with tourniquets. A catheter with separate lumen for the delivery of the cardioplegic solution and venting the aorta is placed in the proximal ascending aorta. The patient is placed on cardiopulmonary bypass and the aorta is cross-clamped. Cardioplegia is delivered to arrest the heart, and cold saline solution is poured over the surface of the heart to topically cool the heart. The pericardial well is continuously irrigated with cold saline to provide topical cooling throughout the period of ischemic arrest.

A This illustration shows the patient oriented with the head at the top of the page with the view directly down into the mediastinum through the midline sternotomy. The aorta is cross-clamped, and cardioplegia has been given. The aortic perfusion cannula is distal to the cross-clamp and the aortic root vent is proximal. The vent is aspirating blood from the aorta and, by extension, from the operative site on the coronary artery. The venous cannula is seen exiting the right atrial appendage. The left internal mammary artery is seen in the upper right of the operative field wrapped in a papaverine-soaked sponge. A silastic vessel loop has been passed around the circumflex marginal artery and placed on gentle traction to help in visualization of the artery and to keep the operative field free of blood. An arteriotomy has been placed distal to the obstructing atherosclerotic lesion. The saphenous vein graft, which will be anastomosed to the circumflex marginal artery, is seen just below the internal mammary artery.

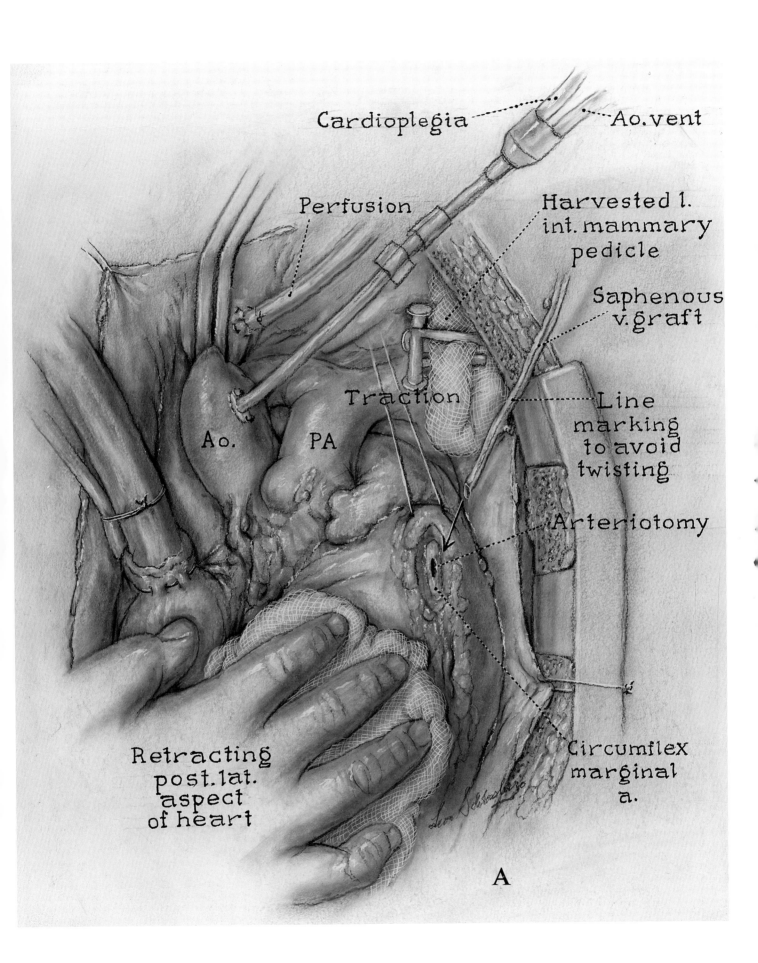

Cardioplegia — Ao.vent

Perfusion

Harvested l. int. mammary pedicle

Saphenous v. graft

Traction

Ao. PA

Line marking to avoid twisting

Arteriotomy

Retracting post.lat. aspect of heart

Circumflex marginal a.

A

B-F The saphenous vein is held by the assistant, and the anastomosis is constructed using a single, continuous 7-0 polypropylene suture. The first three stitches are placed with the saphenous vein held by the assistant above the arteriotomy. The anastomosis is begun at the distal aspect of the arteriotomy to ensure complete visualization and precise suture placement. After the first three sutures are placed, the suture is tightened and the saphenous vein is lowered onto the surface of the heart. The anastomosis continues in a clockwise fashion 360 degrees around the arteriotomy.

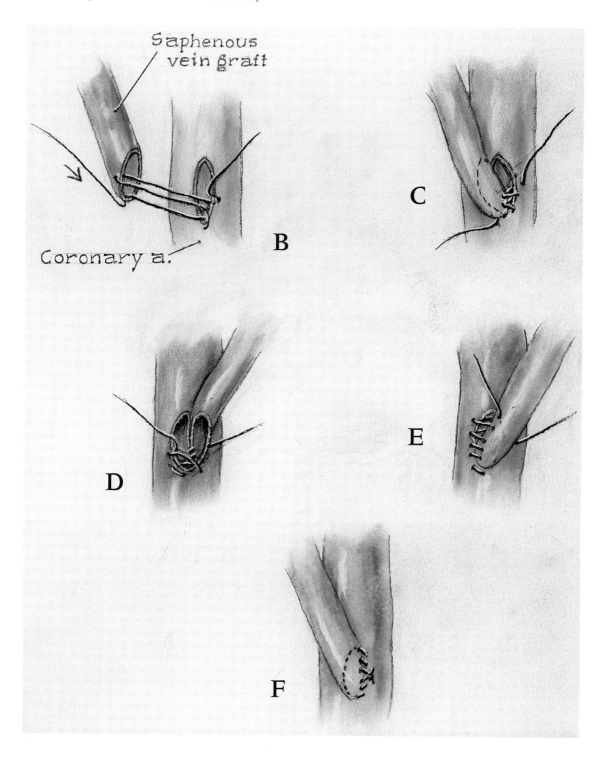

G Once the anastomosis is completed, cardioplegia is delivered into the aortic root and down the vein graft. This is done to check for anastomotic leaks, confirm flow through the graft, assess the proper orientation required of the vein graft, measure the length of vein needed to reach the aorta for the proximal anastomosis, and deliver additional cardioplegia into an area distal to the arterial obstruction.

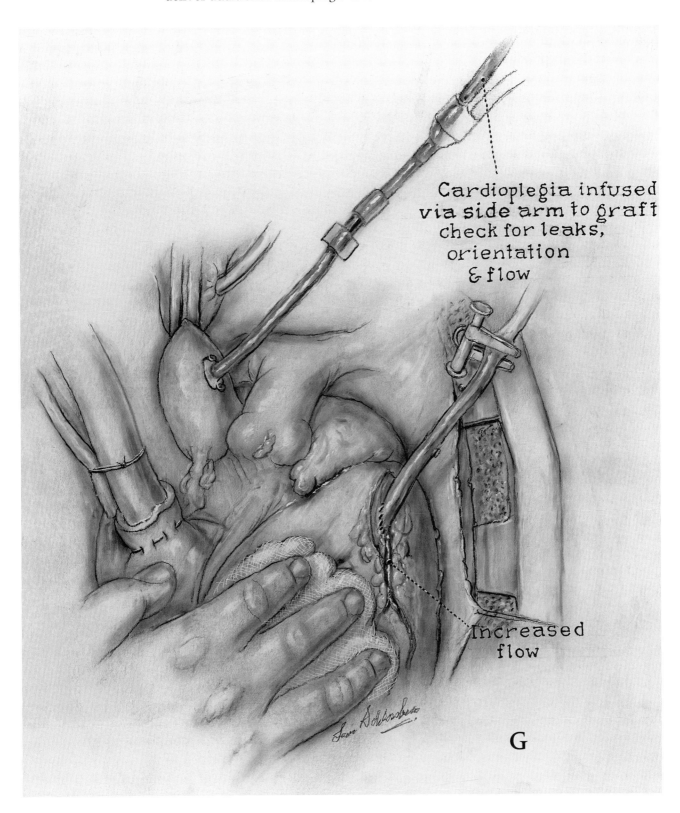

Cardioplegia infused via side arm to graft check for leaks, orientation & flow

Increased flow

G

H The second saphenous vein is anastomosed to the right coronary artery. The heart is positioned, and vessel loops are placed around the right coronary artery. An arteriotomy is created, and the anastomosis is performed as previously described. Visible is the saphenous vein graft to the circumflex marginal coronary artery.

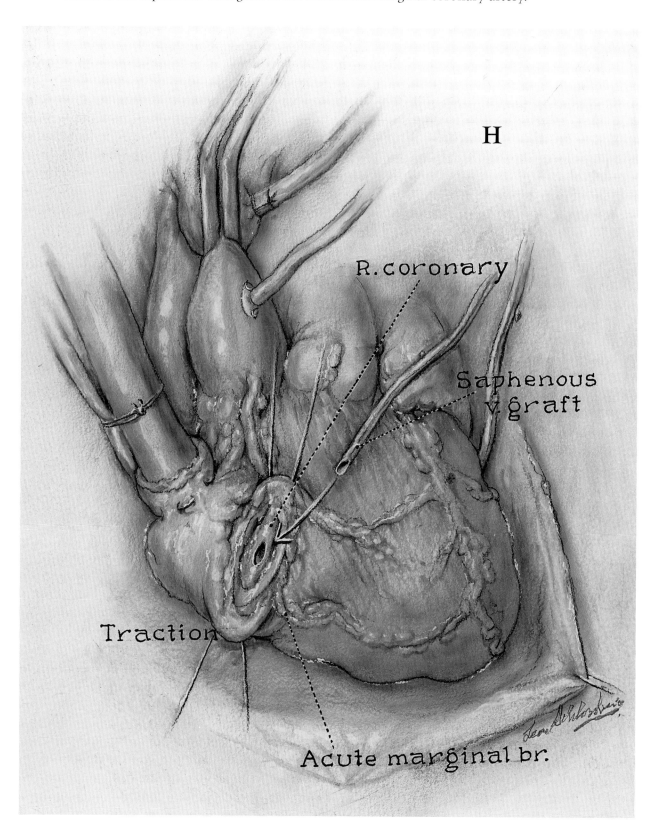

I   The final anastomosis to be completed is the left internal mammary artery to the
left anterior descending coronary artery. The pedicle of the internal mammary
artery is brought into the operative field and prepared for grafting. This consists
of dissecting connective tissue and venous branches off the artery as a preliminary
step. The artery is then grasped by the adventitia and the distal end of the artery
opened obliquely in preparation for anastomosis.

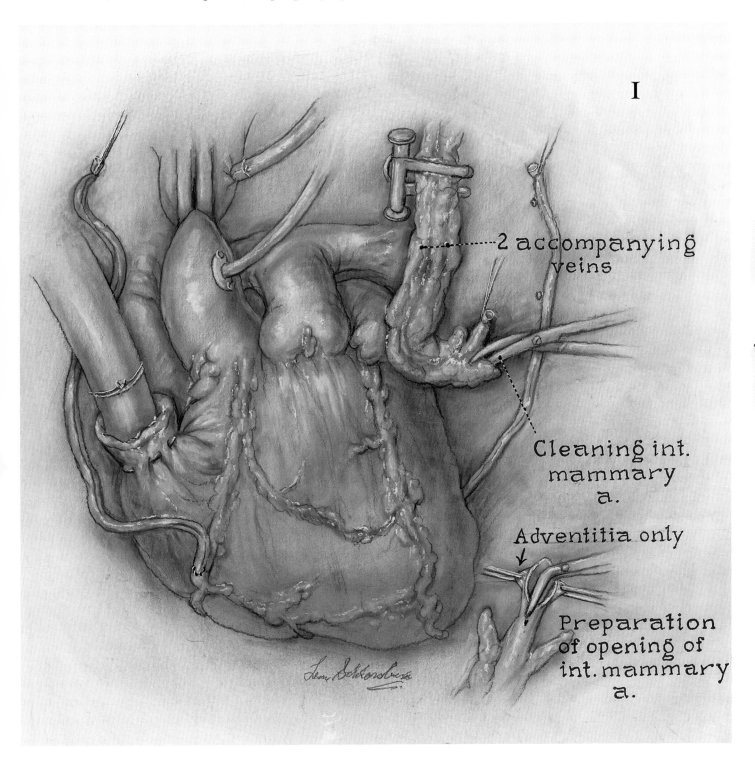

I

2 accompanying veins

Cleaning int. mammary a.

Adventitia only

Preparation of opening of int. mammary a.

J The anastomosis of the internal mammary artery is shown in steps. It is performed in a counterclockwise fashion using a continuous stitch of 7-0 polypropylene suture.

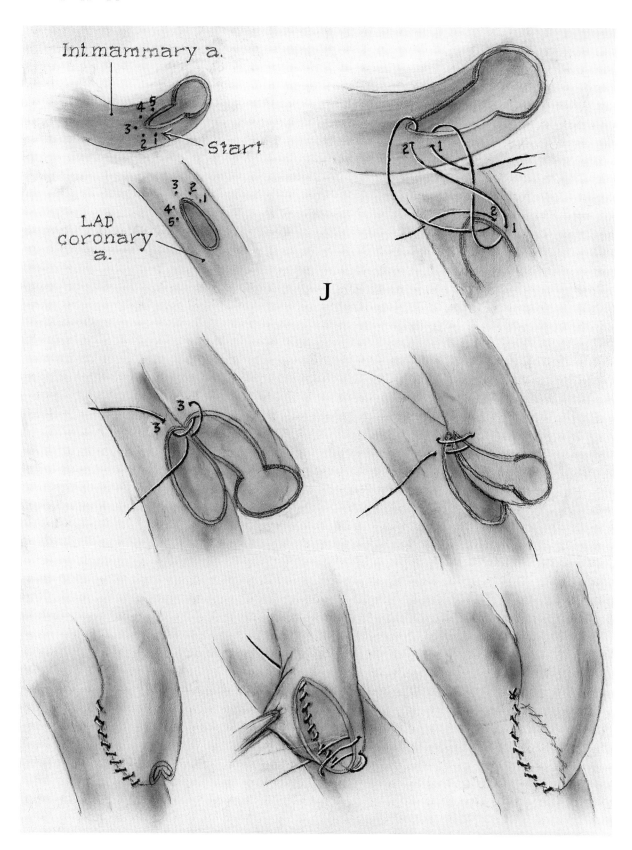

J

K After all of the distal anastomoses are completed, the proximal aortosaphenous anastomoses are constructed. The aortic cross-clamp is removed, and the heart is reperfused through the native circulation and the internal mammary artery. A partial occlusion clamp is placed on the ascending aorta. Aortotomies are created using an aortic punch after an initial incision is made into the aorta at the indicated sites. Care is taken to trim the saphenous veins to the proper length

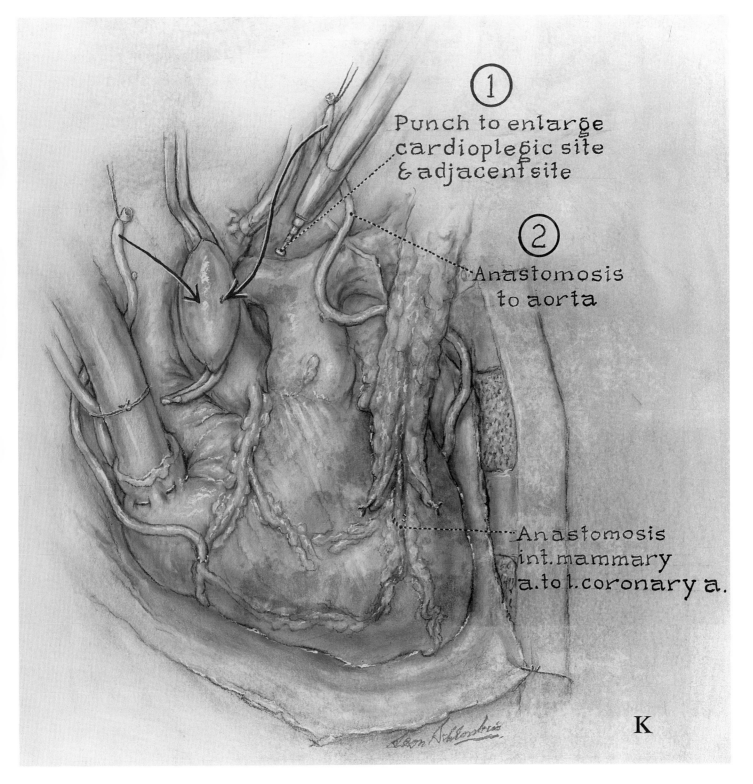

① Punch to enlarge cardioplegic site & adjacent site

② Anastomosis to aorta

Anastomosis int. mammary a. to l. coronary a.

K

prior to constructing the anastomoses. The vein graft to the circumflex marginal graft is routed under the internal mammary artery. A notch is created in the pericardium at the point where the internal mammary artery enters the mediastinum to allow the artery to assume a more medial and inferior position and avoid stretching caused by the inflated lung.

L   The proximal vein graft anastomoses are constructed in an end-to-side fashion using a continuous stitch of 6-0 polypropylene suture.

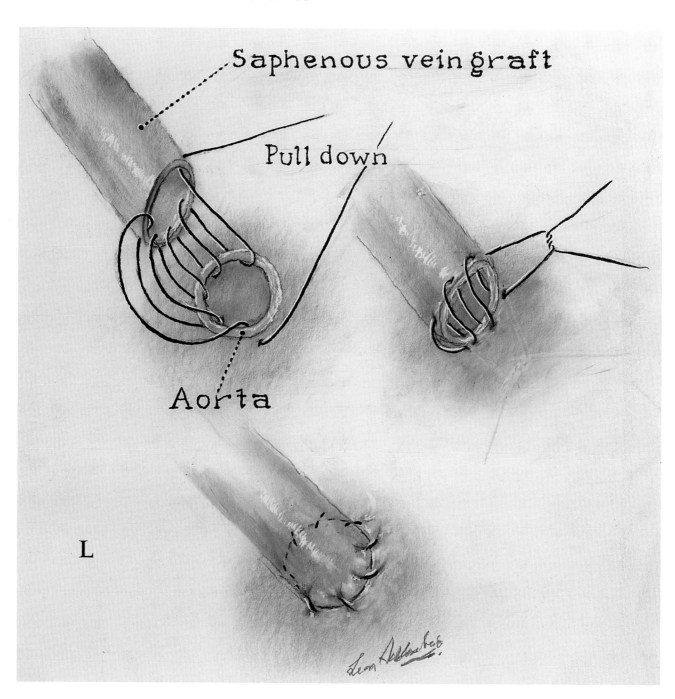

L

M   After the proximal anastomoses are completed, the partial occlusion clamp is
removed. The vein grafts are de-aired with a 25-gauge needle, and the heart is
completely reperfused. The patient is reperfused until ready to be weaned
from bypass.

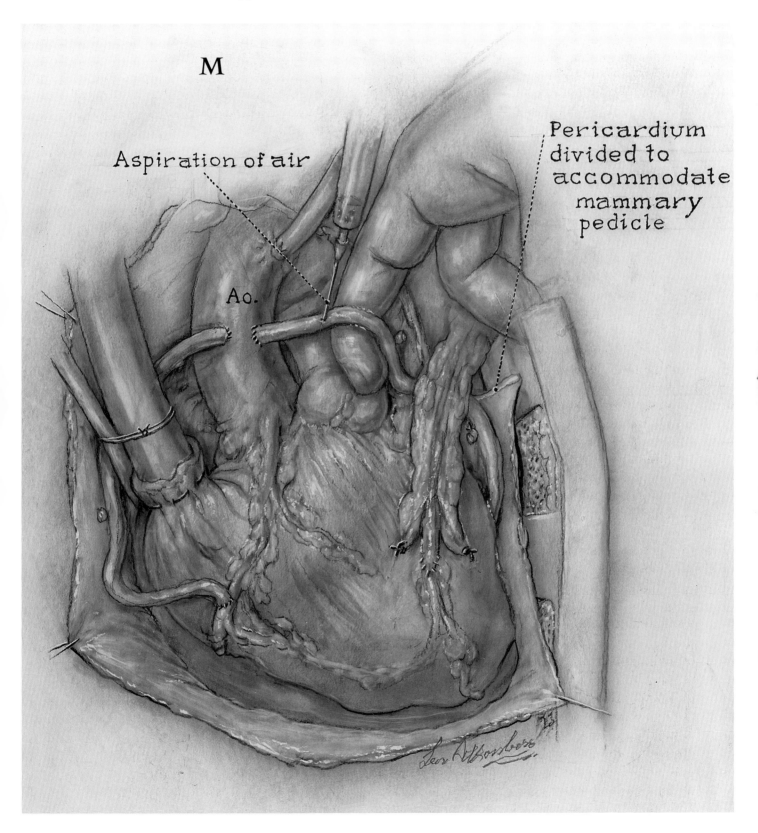

M

Aspiration of air

Ao.

Pericardium
divided to
accommodate
mammary
pedicle

Chapter 3

Port Access Techniques

R. Scott Stuart, M.D.

Introduction

There are many techniques in current cardiac surgery that carry the title Minimally Invasive Cardiac Surgery. The approaches which employ beating heart surgery (MIDCAB, OPCAB) are specifically for, and limited to, coronary artery bypass grafting. Port-access techniques, however, use cardiopulmonary bypass most commonly via the femoral route and employ smaller non-sternotomy incisions to complete the procedure. Since cardiopulmonary bypass is employed, theoretically all cardiac procedures, including those for valve and septal defects, could be approached with this technology. This chapter describes the basic approach for port-access coronary artery bypass grafting via a left anterior thoracotomy and closure of atrial septal defects and the mitral valve approaches via a right anterior thoracotomy.

Port Access Coronary Artery Bypass Grafting

The patient is initially placed in the supine position. The operating room table should be prepared by the placement of a bean bag on the bed. This will facilitate subsequent positioning of the patient after induction of anesthesia. After placing the traditional monitoring, anesthesia is induced and the patient intubated with a double-lumen tube which will allow deflation of the left lung during the operation. Subsequently, an endopulmonary vent (Heartport) is placed into position by advancing the vent over a previously placed Swan-Ganz catheter. This ensures positioning of the pulmonary vent within the main pulmonary artery. The Swan is subsequently removed for the duration of the case. Finally, external defibrillation patches are applied to the back and right anterior chest wall. At this point, the patient is positioned with the chest rotated to elevate the left side as much as possible while keeping the pelvis relatively flat. This position is augmented by engagement of the bean bag and any subsequent padding necessary for the patient's anatomy.

A-B   After appropriate prepping and draping, the original incision is made in the left infrapectoral fold. For women the incision is made in the intramammary fold.

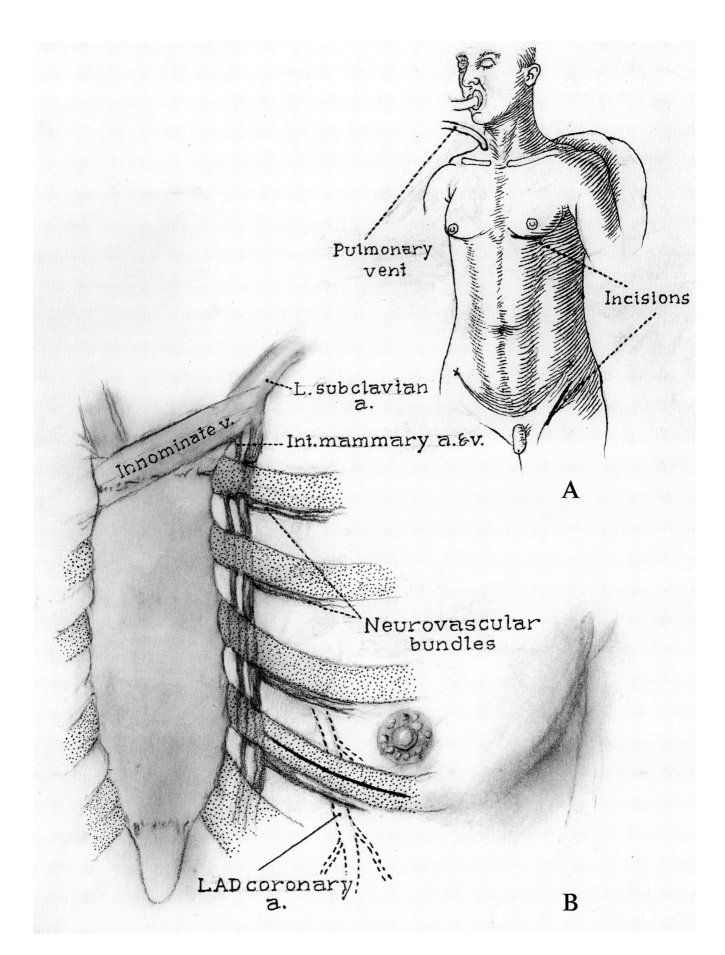

Pulmonary vent

Incisions

A

L. subclavian a.

Innominate v.

Int. mammary a. & v.

Neurovascular bundles

LAD coronary a.

B

C-F The incision is carried down onto the chest wall at a point that overlies the fourth rib (Figure C). The fourth rib and its costal cartilage are exposed and, most frequently, the point of articulation between the fourth costal cartilage and the sternum is divided. This is often performed bluntly, using a large Allis clamp on the costal cartilage and a gentle rocking motion to disengage the costo-sternal junction. In our experience, it is useful to remove the section of the fourth costal cartilage to improve exposure of the underlying mammary artery (Figure D). Once this is performed, the mammary artery itself will be appreciated in the medial aspect of the wound. General dissection of the mammary artery from its bed is then begun with hand-held retraction, which is then rapidly augmented by externally applied devices—either traditional mammary retractors or one of a variety of chest wall elevators which have been specifically designed to facilitate the mammary dissection from this type of incision (Figure E). The mammary artery is then taken down in a fashion similar to the experience in an open chest case, except that the dissection is primarily carried out on the anterior aspect of the artery (Figure F). The dissection is carried up as far superiorly as possible, and frequently this equates to the level of the subclavian vein.

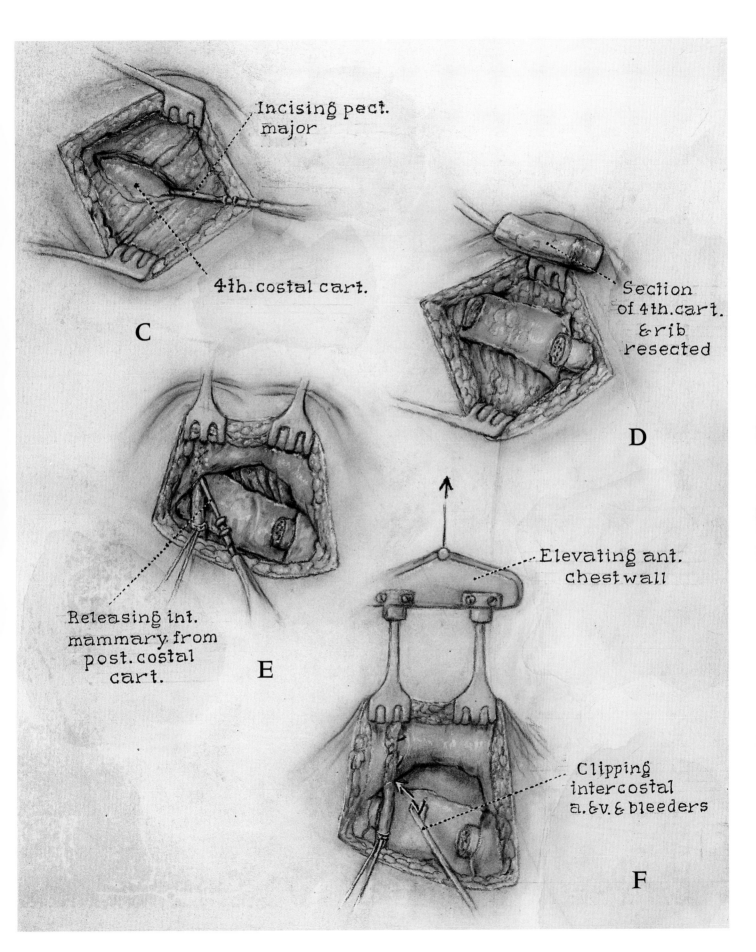

Incising pect. major

4th. costal cart.

C

Section of 4th. cart. & rib resected

D

Releasing int. mammary from post. costal cart.

E

Elevating ant. chest wall

Clipping intercostal a. & v. & bleeders

F

G   Subsequently, attention is turned to gaining distal length of the mammary artery. Most frequently, this is approximately one interspace below the incision due to the limiting nature of the elevated distal chest wall. Once the dissection is completed, 5000 units of heparin are administered and the mammary is divided and prepared for use in the anticipated anastomosis.

H   At this point, attention is turned to the left groin region, where an incision is made in the crease of the left groin for a distance of approximately 5 cm. The common femoral artery and vein are then prepared for use in cardiopulmonary bypass. Frequently, it is easiest to first introduce the venous cannula (DLP #28 French long catheter), which is advanced via the Seldinger technique into the right atrium. The tip of this venous cannula is ideally situated at the junction between the superior vena cava and the right atrium and is confirmed by transesophageal echocardiography. Subsequently, the femoral artery is approached. The arterial catheter (Heartport) is introduced with standard technique. This arterial cannula is unique for its y-shaped design, an arterial inflow aspect, and a side port which contains a screw valve for introduction of the endo clamp. When the arterial cannula is introduced into the artery, it is imperative that both limbs of this cannula are adequately de-aired. Of note, make sure the screw clamp is in the closed position prior to introduction; otherwise the distal surgical field will be appropriately "decorated." With all connections having been made to the bypass circuit, the side port of the arterial inflow catheter is isolated with tubing clamps, and the endoclamp is inserted through the screw valve. Once in place, that valve is closed to ensure homeostasis, but not so tightly as to impinge free advancement of the endoclamp. At this point the tubing clamps on the arterial cannula are removed and the endoclamp is advanced to an appropriate position by the use of a Seldinger technique with the balloon being appropriately positioned in the ascending aorta approximately 2 cm distal to the aortic valve. This position is confirmed with transesophageal echocardiography.

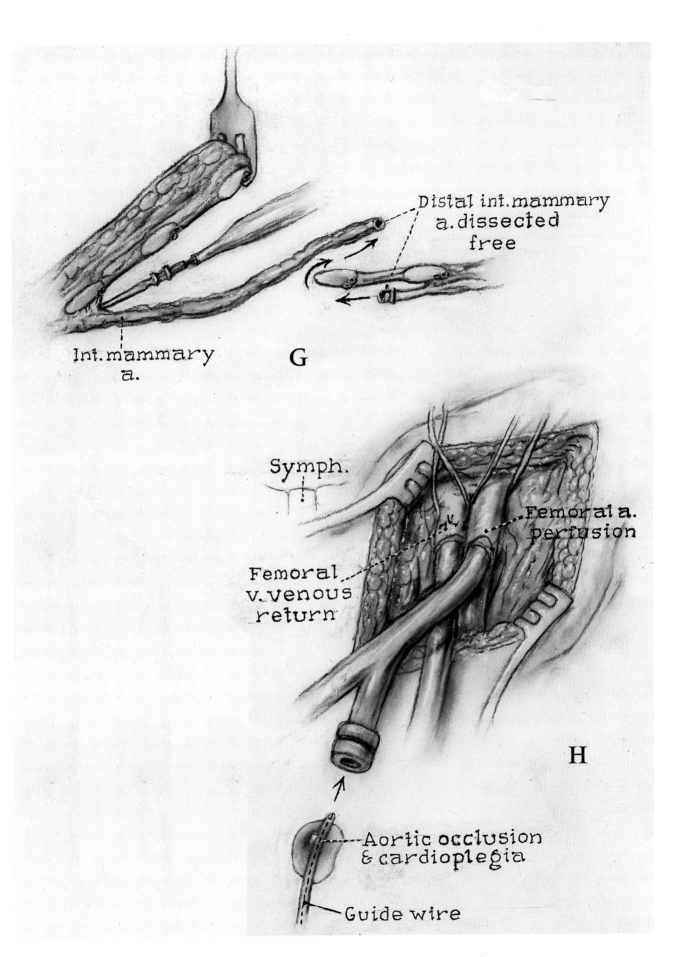

Distal int. mammary
a. dissected
free

Int. mammary
a.

G

Symph.

Femoral a.
perfusion

Femoral
v. venous
return

H

Aortic occlusion
& cardioplegia

Guide wire

I   Next, attention is turned to the pericardium, which is approached through the left thoracotomy. The pericardium is opened extensively with the superior aspect reaching the pulmonary artery and the distal aspect being carried down to just above the diaphragm.

J   The underlying left anterior descending coronary artery should be easily visible, and the mammary artery, which will be used for the subsequent anastomosis, should be positioned within the field. At this point cardiopulmonary bypass is begun and the endoclamp is subsequently inflated. This is done slowly without the cessation of flow through the pump. The endoclamp is fully inflated and its position is confirmed by echocardiography.

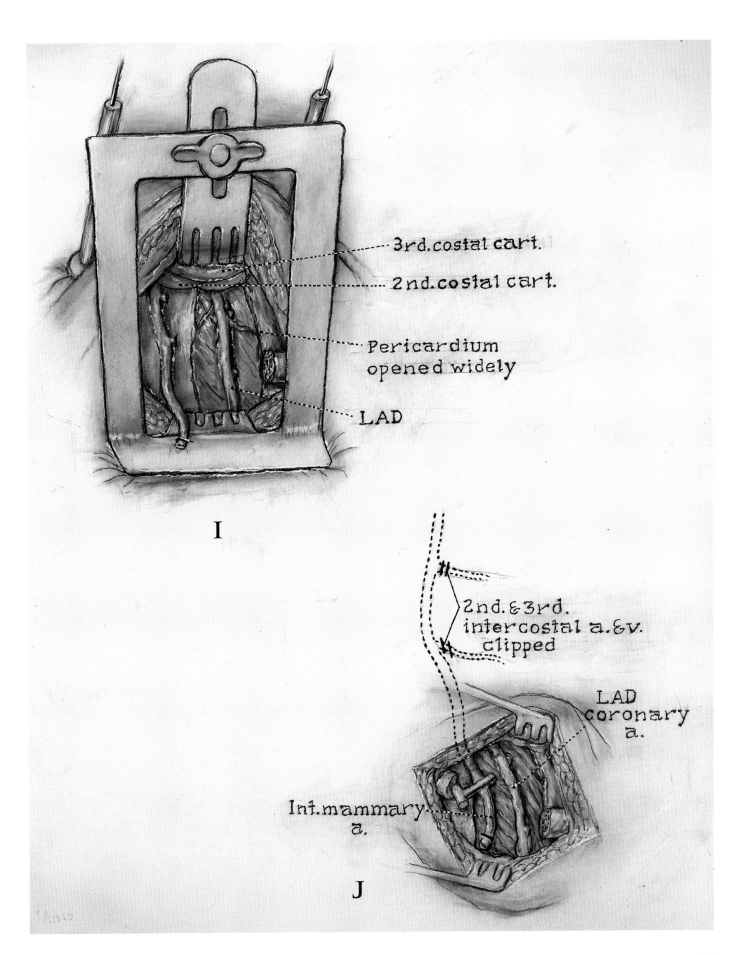

3rd. costal cart.

2nd. costal cart.

Pericardium
opened widely

LAD

I

2nd. & 3rd.
intercostal a. & v.
clipped

LAD
coronary
a.

Int. mammary
a.

J

K The cardioplegia is instilled from the pump via the endoclamp itself.

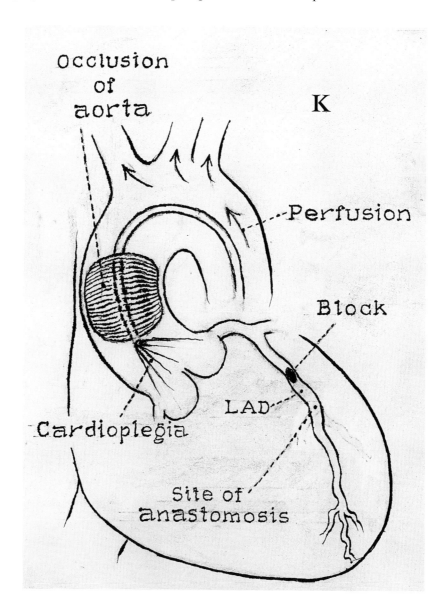

Once electrical silence is obtained, the LAD is isolated, by elastic bands, and a traditional LIMA to LAD anastomosis is performed using either a running 7-0 or 8-0 prolene suture.

At the completion of the anastomosis, the occluding clip is removed from the IMA pedicle to check patency and hemostasis. The endoclamp is then deflated and the entire endoclamp assembly is withdrawn to the side port of the femoral cannula. Of note, when the endoclamp is traversing the cannula itself, flow is temporarily decreased so as not to engender high pump pressures while the endoclamp balloon transits the tip of the arterial cannula. Following the positioning of the endoclamp, the heart is returned to electrical rhythm via external cardioversion, if necessary, and the patient is subsequently weaned from cardiopulmonary bypass. The pericardium is loosely closed over the anastomosis site on the heart, chest tubes are placed within the left pleural space, and the incision is closed in the standard fashion. Of note, we often will place a long epidural catheter within the chest wall. This is positioned so that the tip of the catheter is lying along the medial aspect of the posterior chest wall and superior to the incision. Thus, local anesthesia may be administered as a slow drip in the postoperative period, achieving excellent local anesthesia and minimizing the need for large amounts of narcotics in the postoperative stage. This often allows us to extubate the patient on the operative table if patient age and condition warrant. Finally, the arterial and venous femoral catheters are removed and those vessels repaired with running 5-0 prolene sutures. The groin wound is then closed in the routine fashion.

Port Access Closure of an Atrial Septal Defect

Introduction

The standard approach to the repair of an atrial septal defect (ASD) is via median sternotomy, to cannulate centrally, and to arrest the heart and approach the ASD or patent foramen ovale (PFO) through a right atriotomy. Historically, these lesions were approached via a right anterior thoracotomy with peripheral cannulation for cardiopulmonary bypass or simply by inflow occlusion. The right anterior thoracotomy fell out of favor as median sternotomy gained in popularity. Anterolateral thoracotomy was restricted to use in patients who could not or should not receive a sternotomy, and/or those few patients for whom a cosmetic incision was paramount.

Interest in using various right thoracotomy incisions for approaching ASDs has been renewed in the last few years. With the advent of port access techniques and instruments designed by The Heartport Corporation, this approach allows for a small anterolateral thoracotomy (incision 7–9 cm in length), femoro-femoral cannulation, and the option of using cardiac arrest or fibrillatory arrest.

The patient is brought into the operating room and placed in the supine position. After induction of general anesthesia, intubation is accomplished with a double-lumen endotracheal tube to allow selective deflation of the right lung. The patient is then placed in the modified decubitus position with the right side up (approximately 45 degrees). The hips are left as supine as possible to allow optimal access to the right femoral vessels for use in cardiopulmonary bypass. The patient's position is maintained either by cloth rolls, or preferably by the use of a malleable "bean bag."

Following standard prep and draping procedures, simultaneous incisions are made in the right groin and the right anterior chest wall (Figure A). The groin incision is made in a shallow "S" fashion using the groin fold for most of the incision. A short segment of right femoral artery is prepared in the standard fashion. Our preference for venous cannulation is actually to isolate the saphenous bulb and to divide the greater saphenous vein as it enters the bulb. The bulb itself then receives a purse-string suture of 5-0 prolene, which is placed at its confluence with the common femoral vein. Thus the bulb is used for an appendage cannulation not unlike that of a right atrial appendage.

The right anterolateral thoracotomy is made in the submammary fold for women and the subpectoral crease in men. The incision is carried down to the chest wall where the fourth rib is identified and the third intercostal space entered after deflation of the lung. Neither rib nor cartilage is divided. Prior to extending the third intercostal space incision, a small thoracoscope may be inserted through the original entry into the chest to confirm the incision's position relative to the right atrium. The third intercostal space should be quite satisfactory in gaining a middle position relative to the right atrium. Often the right diaphragm will protrude somewhat into vision, and at this point the third intercostal space incision is extended to approximately 9 cm in length, and the doming diaphragm is handled with the use of a 3-0 prolene suture placed through the dome of the diaphragm in a figure-eight fashion. Retraction is then achieved by passing a 14-gauge angiocath from the external chest wall over the seventh or eighth rib anteriorly and entering the chest cavity, with the exit of the catheter being anterior to the dome of the diaphragm. Through the angiocatheter is inserted a Heartport "crochet needle." With the use of this needle, the 3-0 prolene is withdrawn through the 14-gauge angiocatheter and brought to the outside of the chest wall (Figure C). The dome of the diaphragm is retracted and the suture is externally secured with a rubber snap. A small Finechetto retractor is placed through the thoracotomy incision, and widening of that incision gained through gradual expansion of the retractor.

The pericardium may then be opened with an incision that parallels the phrenic nerve, approximately 1 to 1.5 centimeters superior to the phrenic (Figure B). The pericardium itself is opened from its reflection on the surface of the diaphragm superiorly to the mid portion of the superior vena cava. Its retraction is accomplished with a 3-0 prolene suture placed in a fashion identical to that described for the diaphragmatic retraction. Tension is placed on the sutures as they are brought laterally and are passed over the top of the fifth and third ribs. Retraction of the anterior aspect of the pericardium may be accomplished through the superior aspect of the thoracotomy incision. Excellent exposure of the right atrium should be obtained at this time.

The next move is to gain access around both the inferior and superior vena cavae. The standard dissection is undertaken and is actually quite simple with this approach. Rumel tourniquets are placed around the inferior and superior vena cavae in the standard fashion using a Semb clamp. Cannulation of the superior vena cava may be accomplished directly with the use of a right-angled cannula, but most frequently we have preferred to approach the SVC cannulation via the right atrial appendage. At this point we have traditionally placed a standard right atrial appendage purse-string cannulation suture. Heparin is administered and cannulation is performed via the common femoral vessels. The vein is most easily cannulated first; as implied above, this is done using a DLP #28

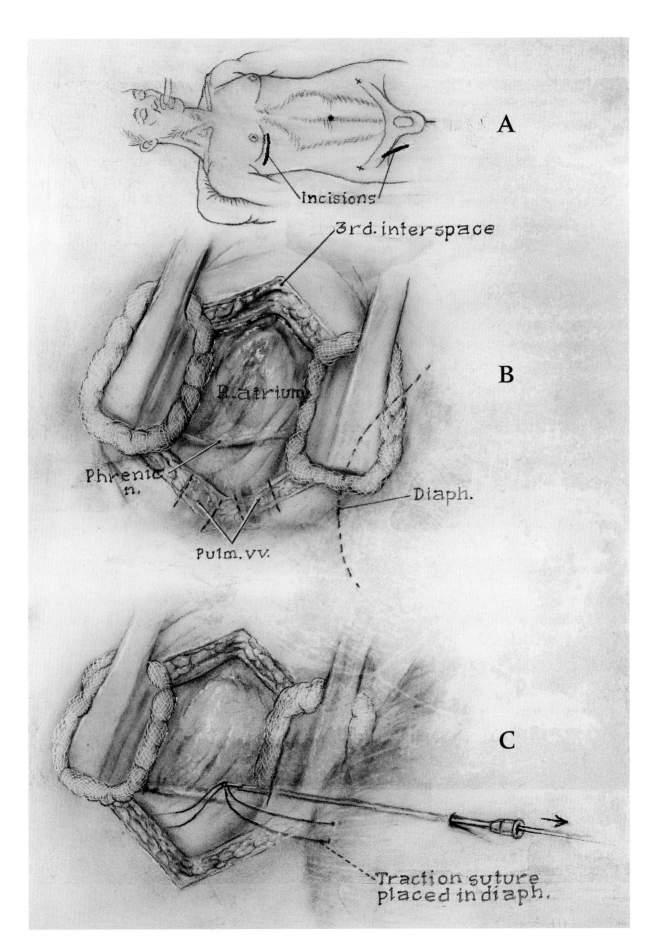

A

Incisions

3rd. interspace

B

R.atrium

Phrenic
n.

Pulm. vv.

Diaph.

C

Traction suture
placed in diaph.

French catheter via a Seldinger technique. The catheter is passed through the saphenous bulb, and a keeper on the purse-string suture at the base of the bulb allows for variable position of the venous catheter as well as security of the catheter within the femoral vein. Its position should be within the intrahepatic IVC and palpably confirmed by advancing the catheter tip into the right atrium until felt by a probing finger, then withdrawn an appropriate length to ensure that the tip is within the intrahepatic IVC. In turn, arterial cannulation via the right common femoral artery is performed in the standard fashion.

Attention is then turned to the right atrium, where most commonly a #28 French catheter is placed via the right atrial appendage and advanced into the superior vena cava. We have found that the ease of placement of this cannula is markedly enhanced by inserting a sterile endotracheal tube guide into the #28 catheter, thus facilitating "intubation" of the superior vena cava via the right atrial appendage. Bypass is then initiated, and traditionally we cool the patient to 32 degrees centigrade. Temporary pacing wires of the alligator variety are placed on the anterior surface of the right ventricle (which is easily approached through this incision) and a fibrillator box employed to induce ventricular fibrillation.

Once this is achieved, both Rumel tourniquets are engaged and the right atrium is opened with a vertical incision. Regional infusion of CO_2 is now started at 7 L/min. The coronary sinus return can easily be controlled by the placement of a small vent within the orifice of the coronary sinus. At this point the fossa ovale with its PFO, or the ASD, should be easily appreciated. The level of blood in the field is controlled with a pump sucker so that the left atrial level is as high as possible to minimize introduction of air into the left atrium. The PFO is closed in the standard fashion with individual sutures of 4-0 prolene. The ASD is closed either by primary closure using 4-0 prolene or, if the ASD is large enough, we will use a patch closure with native pericardium which has been cut to size (Figure D). Such a patch will traditionally be anchored in 3 or 4 positions with a 4-0 prolene suture, and the intervening closure between the septal defect and patch is performed with a running 4-0 suture (Figure F). Knot tying is facilitated using a Heartport knot-pusher (Figure E). Again, much of this closure is done nearly "underwater" to minimize introduction of air into the left atrium.

After completion of the ASD repair, the right atriotomy is closed with a 3-0 prolene suture. The Rumel tourniquets are released and the left atrium is inspected for air using transesophageal echo. If no air is appreciated (which is the rule) the heart is defibrillated using external Zohl patches. If air is noticed within the left atrium, de-airing may be carried out by placing a small de-airing catheter in the root of the aorta, which is easily approached through this incision.

With the patient in the decubitus position, the right lateral aspect of the aorta will become the highest point in the aorta, and the de-airing is carried out after the patient has been placed in Trendelenburg position. The patient is then weaned from cardiopulmonary bypass, and groin decannulation is accomplished. The saphenous bulb is easily controlled by simply tying off the 5-0 prolene suture. Likewise, the right atrial appendage is closed with ligation of the purse-string suture. Protamine is administered and the chest wound is closed in layers. We have been using #2 pericostal stitches despite not having to divide the ribs, since they are often bowed from the retractor by the end of the

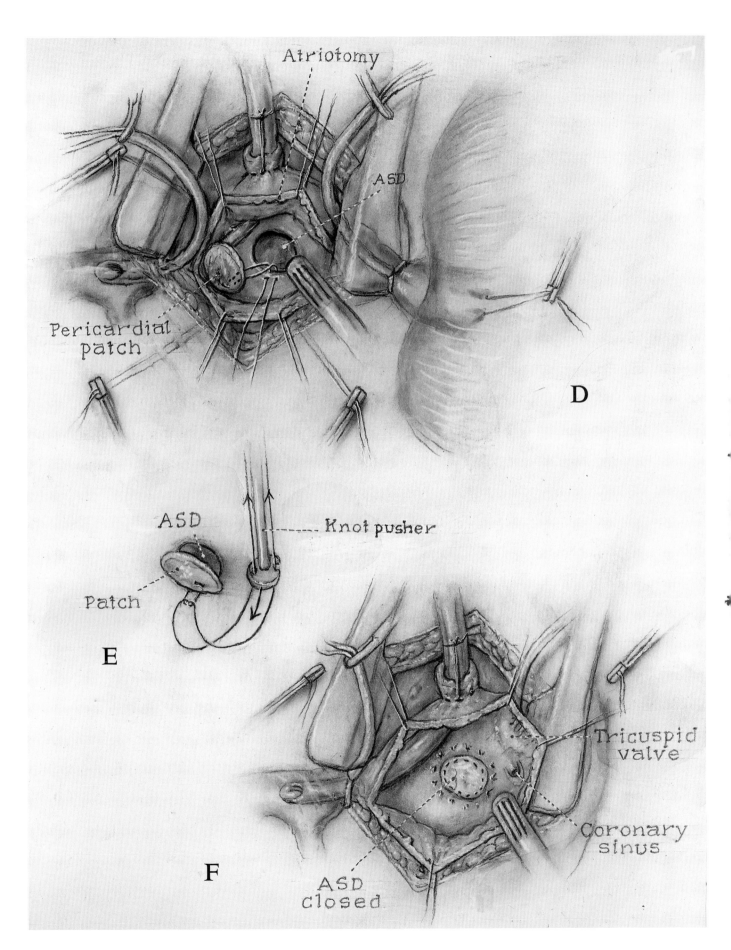

Atriotomy

ASD

Pericardial
patch

D

ASD

Knot pusher

Patch

E

Tricuspid
valve

Coronary
sinus

ASD
closed

F

procedure. The patient may be extubated on the table if the procedure has been brief and the patient is young, or changing to a single lumen tube may be considered at this time by anesthesia should continued intubation be required. If there are any concerns with airway edema, the double lumen tube is left in place and both lungs ventilated.

This procedure may also be performed using cardiac arrest via the Heartport Endo-clamp. This is placed through the side port of the arterial cannula as supplied by the Heartport Corporation. It position may be confirmed by either TE echo or fluoroscopy. If employing the endo-clamp, it is recommended that bilateral radial arterial lines be placed in order to monitor possible distal balloon migration, which would present itself as a diminution in the right radial pressure compared to left radial pressure. When cardio-plegic arrest is used, air is virtually always introduced into the left atrium, and de-airing maneuvers are necessary. Again, this may be done directly via the use of the aortic root site. Alternatively, some centers have reported success in using the endo-clamp itself, with the endo-clamp balloon deflated at the end of the procedure and then reinflated at approximately one quarter its full size. The position that is assumed will be higher in the aorta, and the central lumen of the endo-clamp can be placed on suction and thus used as an internal de-airing vent. Again, its position and effectiveness can be confirmed with TE echo.

Chapter 4

Left Ventricle Aneurysmorraphy and Postinfarction Ventricular Septal Defects

R. Scott Stuart, M.D.

Left Ventricle Aneurysmorraphy

Left ventricular aneurysms result from a gradual thinning and dilatation of a previous transmural myocardial infarction. They require surgical attention when a patient experiences symptoms of the classic triad: angina of non-CAD origin, recurrent emboli from a thrombotic source in the aneurysm, or congestive heart failure engendered by deterioration in pump efficiency. An overwhelming majority of these aneurysms are anterior in location. Inferior posterior infarctions rarely expand to become clinically significant aneurysms. There are three basic approaches to the repair of an LV aneurysm and each will be discussed in turn.

Left Ventricle Aneurysmorraphy *continued*

A The approach to an LV aneurysm repair begins with standard sternotomy and standard cannulation for cardiopulmonary bypass. Frequently, the aorta is cross-clamped to facilitate technical manipulation of the heart; however, this is not strictly necessary as long as the aortic valve is competent. Once cardiopulmonary bypass is instituted (with or without cross-clamping) attention is turned to the LV aneurysm itself. As illustrated, the extent of the aneurysm will be quite obvious after institution of bypass. The affected area of the left ventricle will become concave. This area is grasped with forceps and resected as shown. A small rim of scar tissue is left to facilitate closure and to avoid the placement of sutures through viable myocardium.

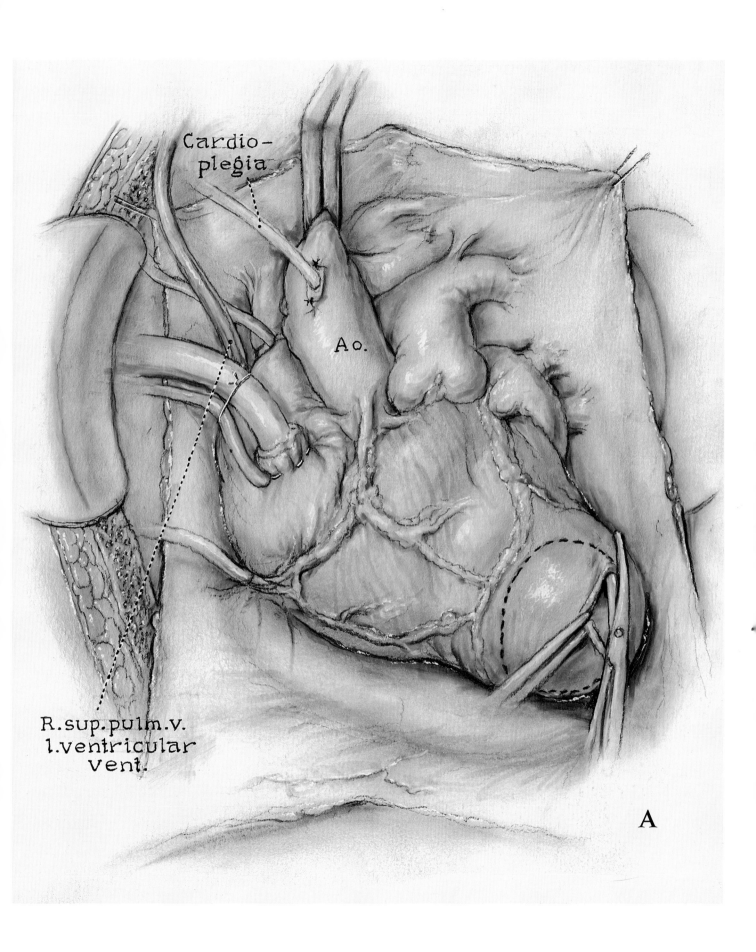

Cardio-
plegia

Ao.

R.sup.pulm.v.
l.ventricular
vent.

A

Left Ventricle Aneurysmorraphy *continued*

B-D After the aneurysmal wall is resected, the left ventricle is inspected for chronic thrombus. Any thrombus found is removed. Subsequently, two strips of reinforcing material (which may be created out of felt or even long strips of native pericardium) are laid out on either side of the open aneurysm, and interrupted mattress sutures of 2-0 or 3-0 prolene are placed across the defect, using the strips as bolsters. After the sutures are placed, they are tied, and a second suture is used (in a running fashion) to hemostatically seal the everted edges.

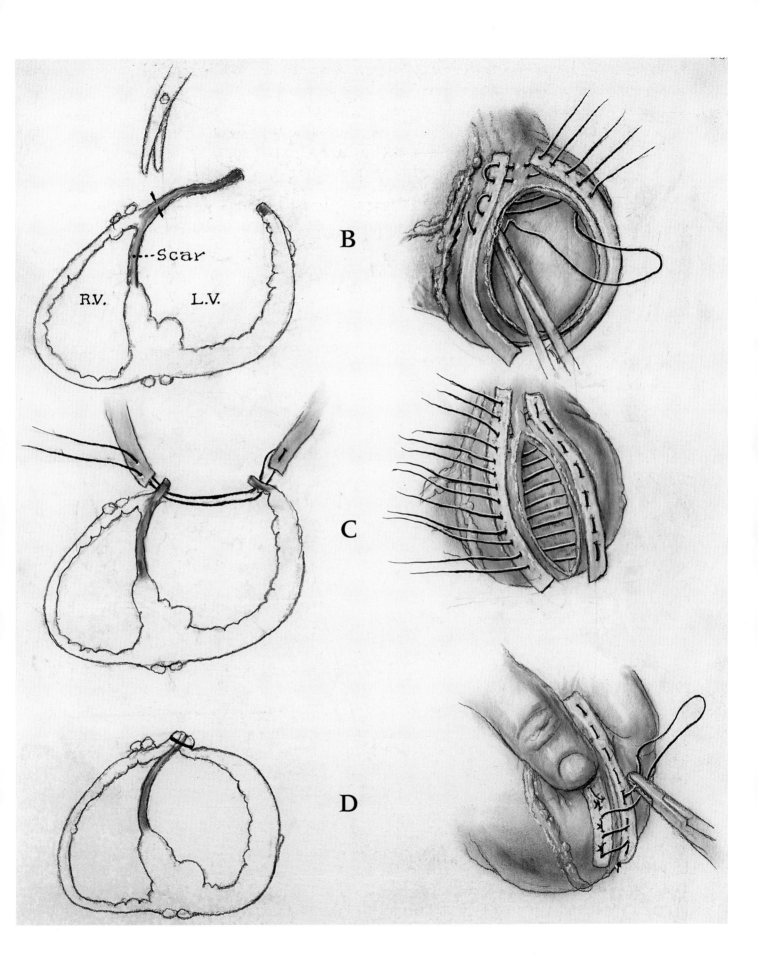

B

C

D

R.V.

L.V.

--Scar

Left Ventricle Aneurysmorraphy *continued*

E The second legitimate approach involves opening the infarct area as described above; however, instead of closing the defect with a vertical suture line, a piece of impervious woven dacron is brought onto the field and an oblong piece fashioned to fit over the defect in the left ventricular free wall. The size of this patch is approximately 3 to 4 millimeters greater than the defect. It is sewn into place with either interrupted mattress sutures of 2-0 ticron or prolene or, alternatively, secured with a running mattress suture. As this patch is closed, volume is taken into the left ventricle, and any air present in the left ventricular cavity is expelled. Any leak in the closure may easily be repaired, since the margin of the graft and left ventricular wall is everted.

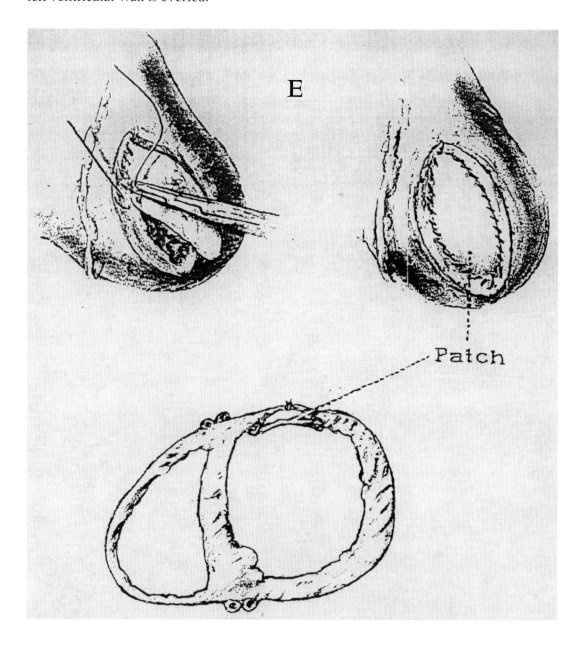

F The last form of repair is a variation of the above technique; however, the aneurysm itself is opened with a single vertically oriented incision and after inspection of the LV cavity a piece of flexible graft material (our preference is a Savage graft) is cut to fit the diameter of the neck of the aneurysm. This area is clearly defined as a fibrous line between the area of the infarct and the normal endocardium. The patch is 2–3 millimeters larger than the actually desired circumference; it is placed within the LV cavity and its edges are sewn to the infarct/aneurysm margin. This is usually performed with a running 3-0 prolene suture. At the completion of this suture line, the still intact aneurysmal sac is closed over the repair patch, usually with a running 3-0 or 4-0 prolene suture. Such a closure has been championed by both Dr. Denton Cooley and Dr. Tirone David and has the advantage of excluding all artificial material from the pericardial space.

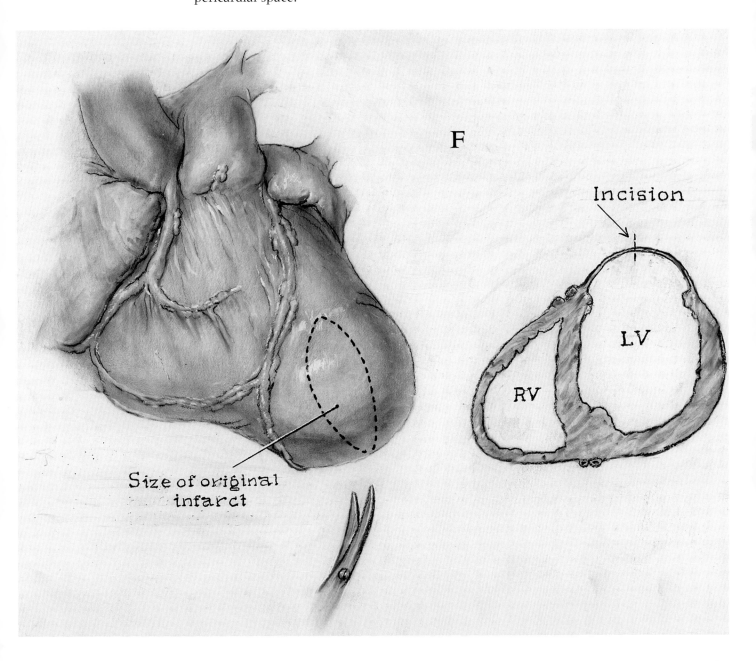

F

Incision

LV

RV

Size of original
infarct

Postinfarction Ventricular Septal Defects

Postinfarction ventricular septal defects are one of the few true cardiac surgical emergencies. Mortality figures are usually fairly high given the nature of the defect and the fact that it is usually occurring within one to five days of a fresh transmural infarction. Over the last several years, the incidence of postinfarction VSDs has seemed to decrease, perhaps due to the widespread use of thrombotic therapy in acute infarction. It is one of the more challenging surgical cases.

A-B One first approaches the VSD through the infarcted aspect of the free wall of the left ventricle. Shown here is a ventriculotomy in the anterior left ventricle with the underlining ventricular septal defect easily appreciated. The VSD is first closed with an independent patch of dacron or Savage. The procedure is begun by placing an individual pledgeted suture within the ventricular septal defect itself. The placement of these sutures is from the left ventricular, through the septum, back via the VSD, and passed through the patch as shown in the illustration. Alternatively, these sutures may be placed with the pledgets within the right ventricular aspect of the septum, brought through the septum and through the patch, thus creating a "boiler plate" type of closure.

C-D The vertical orientation of such a patch is illustrated in this figure. The patch itself is large enough to extend through the ventriculotomy as shown and is subsequently incorporated in a vertical closure of the ventriculotomy, which uses interrupted 2-0 or 3-0 prolene sutures over felt strips. Such a closure is virtually identical to that described in Figures B-D of the previous section.

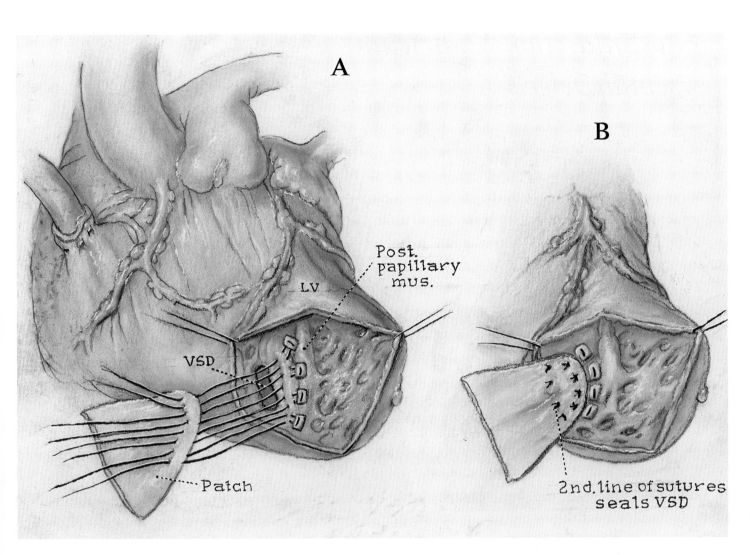

A

B

Post.
papillary
mus.

LV

VSD

Patch

2nd. line of sutures
seals VSD

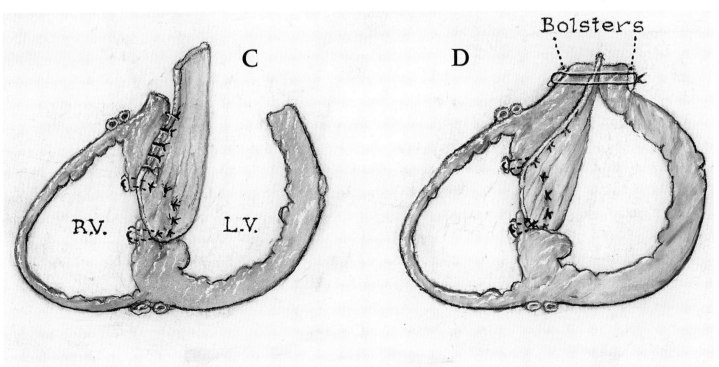

Bolsters

C

D

R.V.

L.V.

Postinfarction Ventricular Septal Defects *continued*

E   Inferior postinfarction VSDs present a more challenging situation and indeed do
     carry a higher mortality. Frequently, a segment of the right ventricle is involved,
     and this contributes to the increased morbidity and mortality with this type of
     infarction. The surgical approach to posterior VSDs is similar in concept to that of
     the anterior VSDs in that a vertical incision is made parallel to the septum and
     through the transmural infarction. As illustrated, most of these infarctions are due
     to closure of the posterior descending coronary system whether it arises from the
     right coronary artery or the circumflex system.

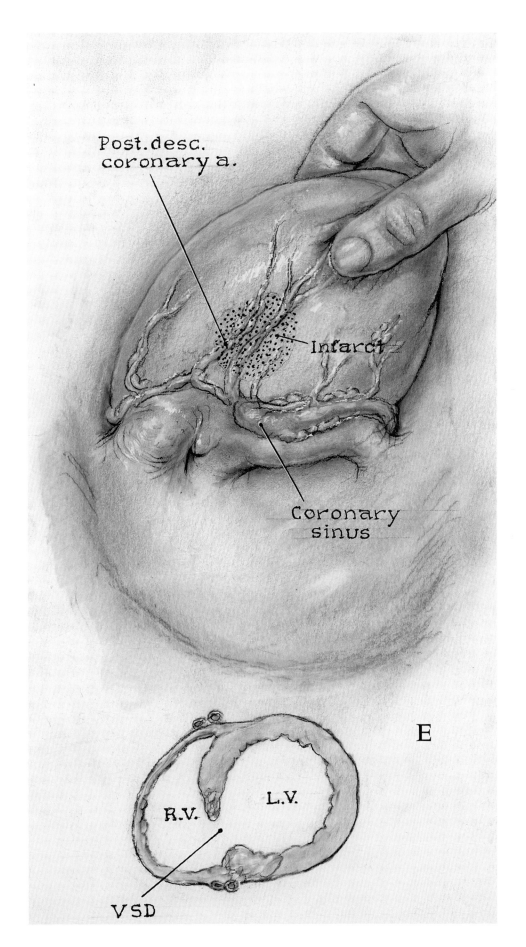

Post. desc.
coronary a.

Infarct

Coronary
sinus

E

L.V.

R.V.

VSD

Postinfarction Ventricular Septal Defects *continued*

F-H This figure depicts the resection of the infarcted tissue surrounding the VSD itself. Some resection is required to enable subsequent technical placement of the interrupted pledgeted sutures. Large resections should not be carried out because this simply creates a larger VSD and places more tension on the patch repair itself. However, it should be noted that the placement of the individual pledgeted sutures must account for the fact that there is always a fairly wide zone of infarction around the VSD itself. If wide enough placement is not accomplished, one runs the risks of subsequent necrosis and peri-patch leak one to three days postoperatively. As shown, the inferior aspect of the pledgeted sutures is first placed with pledgets positioned within the right ventricular cavity. These sutures are then passed through the inferior aspect of the patch, the patch is brought down into the LV cavity, and those sutures are tied. The end sutures for that patch and the subsequent anterior suture line are then positioned with the sutures first being placed through the patch, then through the VSD itself, and brought out through the free wall surface of the ventricle. Those sutures are subsequently tied and the VSD thus closed. It is very difficult to close the ventriculotomy of an inferior infarct using a vertical pledgeted suture line. Therefore, the inferior ventriculotomy is closed with a separate patch in a fashion similar to that described in the second option for aneurysm closure (Figure E in the Left Ventricle Aneurysmorraphy section of this chapter).

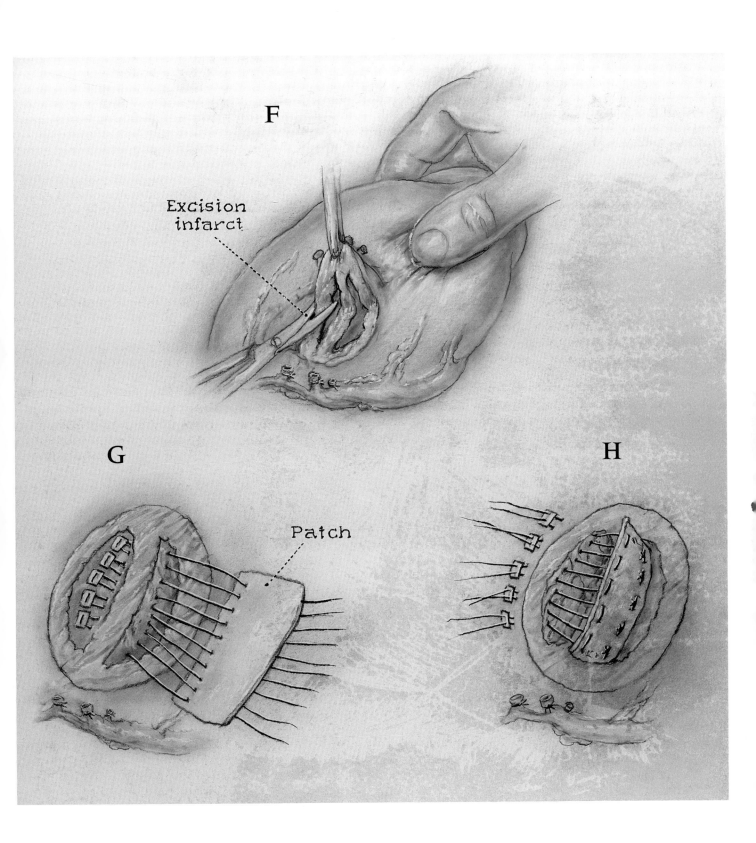

F

Excision
infarct

G

Patch

H

Postinfarction Ventricular Septal Defects *continued*

I-K Occasionally, a left ventricular infarct will affect a papillary muscle and subsequently cause postinfarction mitral regurgitation. In the immediate postinfarct period, such a complication usually presents as pure mitral regurgitation, and the valve replacement is carried out as one would carry out any mitral replacement as described in The Mitral Valve chapter. However, on occasion mitral regurgitation may be combined with a postinfarction ventricular septal defect or may present as a late complication in association with a large left ventricular aneurysm. In either case, the opportunity presents itself to replace the mitral valve through the subsequent left ventriculotomy. This illustration depicts such an approach, with the left ventriculotomy made and the chordae divided at the head of the papillary muscles. The remainder of the mitral apparatus is resected, and individual mattress sutures using pledgets are placed through the mitral annulus in a "boiler plate" fashion. The valve is lowered into place, and seating is ensured as the sutures are tied. Subsequent handling of the ventricular septal defect and/or ventriculotomy closure is carried out as described above. Though these figures show a close relationship of the ventriculotomy to the valve, the infarct and ventriculotomy frequently are fairly distal on the left ventricular surface, and one should be aware that the replacement of the valve often requires longer instruments. The distance between the infarct and the mitral annulus can actually be 2–4 centimeters.

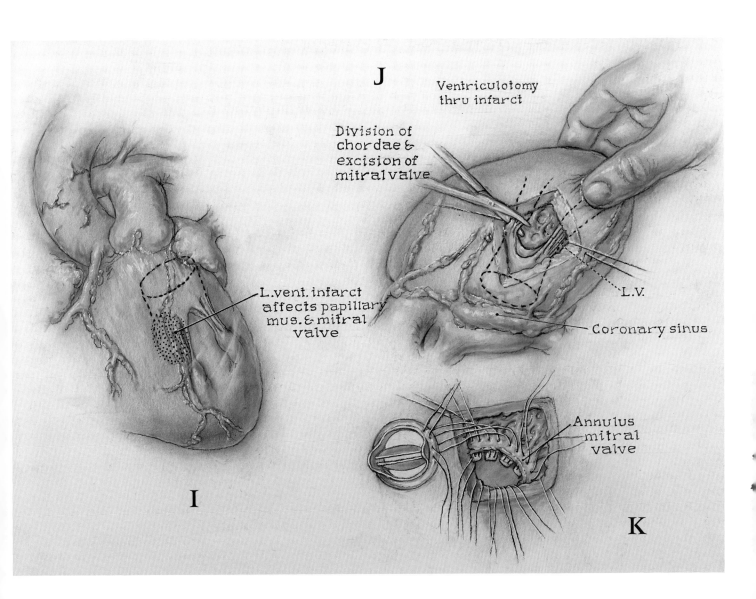

J

Ventriculotomy thru infarct

Division of chordae & excision of mitral valve

L.V.

Coronary sinus

L.vent. infarct affects papillary mus.& mitral valve

I

Annulus mitral valve

K

Postinfarction Ventricular Septal Defects *continued*

L-N The final variation on dealing with a postinfarct ventricular septal defect is that popularized by Tirone David from Toronto. It may be used in either anterior or inferior infarctions with their attendant ventricular septal defects; however, it is most easily used with anterior infarctions. As described earlier, the VSD is originally approached through a left ventriculotomy made in the zone of infarction. If the patient is presenting relatively late following the infarction, there is the possibility an attendant LV aneurysm will be in place as depicted here in Figure L. As previously described, the VSD is inspected, as is the extent of the infarction. An estimate is gained of the extent of the infarct and the compromised myocardium surrounding the VSD itself as seen in Figure M. In this approach, instead of using a separate patch for the VSD and the subsequent ventriculotomy closure, a single large patch is fashioned. It is usually circular or elliptical. The true difference of this approach is that the patch is first placed completely within the left ventricular cavity with the bulk of the patch advanced toward the base of the heart and the mitral valve. Subsequently, the free edge of the patch is sutured with a running 3-0 or 4-0 prolene suture to the **normal** endocardium in a circular line which parallels a demarcation between normal endocardium and infarcted myocardium. When the ventricle ultimately fills with blood, the bulk of the patch material will descend into the lower ventricular cavity (like a windsock) and, since it is attached to normal endocardium, will effectively exclude the entire infarct zone and ventricular septal defect. The increased left ventricular pressure will ensure that the patch will expand and remain in place as implied in Figure N. After the patch placement is completed, the ventriculotomy is closed primarily with a running 3-0 prolene suture. The advantage of such an approach is that the fragile tissue of the infarct and VSD is completely excluded from direct ventricular pressure, and this is a much faster method of VSD closure compared to the independent VSD patch technique. Finally, it should be remembered that, postoperatively, all of these patients will benefit from an intra-aortic balloon pump.

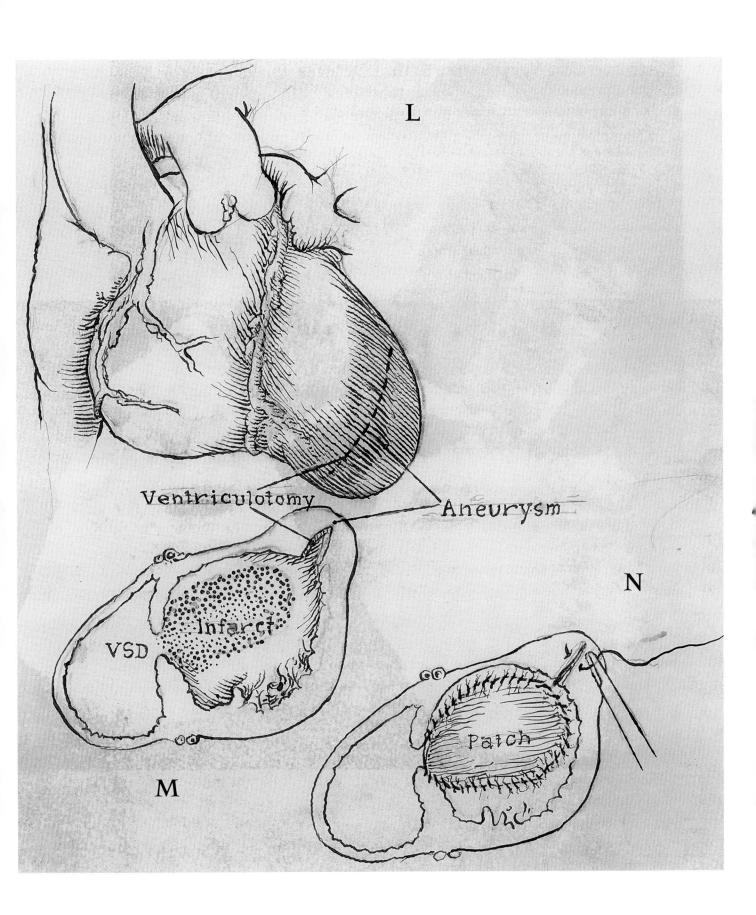

L

Ventriculotomy

Aneurysm

VSD

Infarct

M

Patch

N

Chapter 5

Ventricular Assist Devices

John V. Conte, M.D.

Introduction

Ventricular assist devices are mechanical pumps which can be inserted into a patient's heart to provide circulatory assistance. They can be grouped into two broad categories based upon the duration of circulatory support required. Short-term devices are used to support the circulation until the patient's heart recovers enough to independently support the circulation. These devices may be placed in the setting of an operation in which the patient is unable to be weaned from cardiopulmonary bypass or in the setting of an acute insult, such as a myocardial infarction or acute viral myocarditis, in which the native heart is expected to recover. In contradistinction, long-term devices are used when there is no expectation of native heart recovery. Devices in this situation are intended to be used as a bridge to transplantation while a suitable donor heart is sought. Recently, long-term devices have been applied as destination therapy in which there is no expectation of heart transplantation and no expectation of native heart recovery.

Mechanical circulatory support is a dynamic and evolving field with many devices available or under development, each with its own unique characteristics. Devices can be placed intracorporeally with electrical or pneumatic drive lines connected by transcutaneous routes to the power source. They can also be paracorporeal or extracorporeal, with inflow and outflow conduits exiting the body to pumps resting on or immediately adjacent to the body and connected by drive lines of variable lengths to the power source. Blood flow can be pulsatile or laminar, and the power source can be AC or DC. In pulsatile devices, the pusher plates which cause the ejection of blood from the devices may be mechanical or air driven.

Circulatory support can be univentricular or biventricular. In acute settings, biventricular support is common; in chronic settings, left ventricular assist devices are all that is usually required for circulatory support, although many patients who will require chronic support will require biventricular support for short periods. Mechanical devices designed for short-term use are more likely to be used for biventricular support, whereas the long-term devices are generally used only for left ventricular support.

In the figures in this chapter, the left ventricular assist device depicted is an example of a mechanical, intracorporeal device connected to its power source by a transcutaneous drive line. The patient is oriented with the head to the top and the feet to the bottom of the page.

A   The approach shown is through a midline sternotomy incision. The incision is continued down to the umbilicus. The peritoneal cavity is not breached and a pocket is created in the subcostal region posterior to the rectus muscle, anterior to the posterior rectus sheath, to accommodate placement of the mechanical pump. The patient is placed on cardiopulmonary bypass with standard arterial and venous cannulation. A communication is created through the pericardium and diaphragm into the subcostal space through which the inflow conduit to the pump will be placed. The length of the outflow conduit is measured and anastomosed to the ascending aorta. The insert in the lower left depicts the direction of flow as if it would pass through an aortic valve.

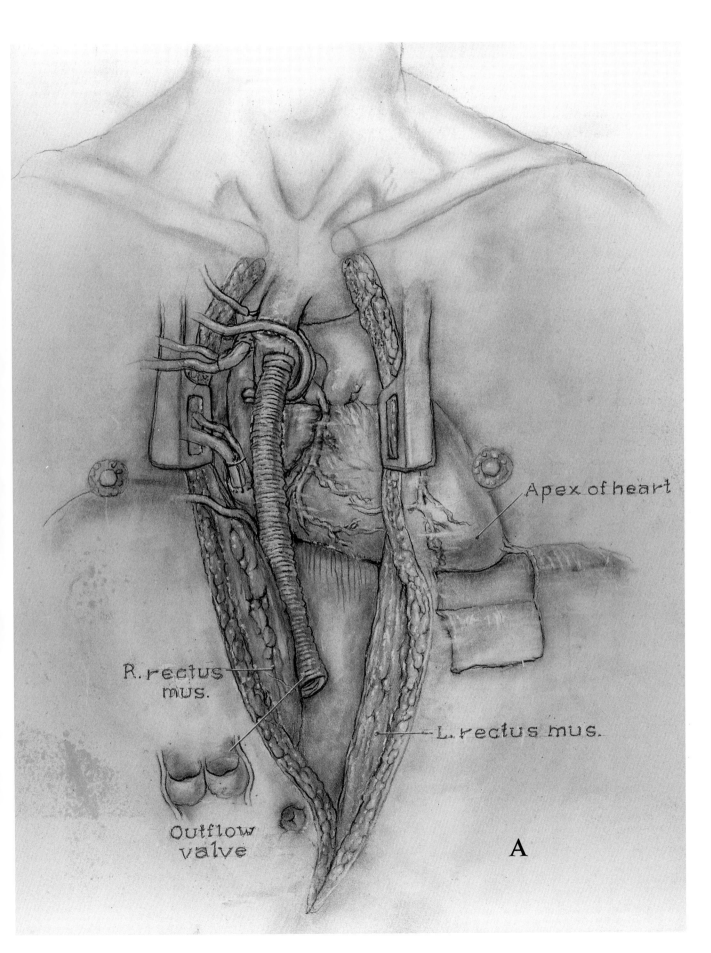

Outflow
valve

R. rectus
mus.

L. rectus mus.

Apex of heart

A

B   A circular opening into the left ventricle is created by excising a portion of the left ventricular apex. The inflow cannula of the pump is passed from the subcostal pocket through the opening in the diaphragm and pericardium and inserted into the left ventricular cavity. This will allow blood to flow out of the left ventricle, providing the inflow to the mechanical pump.

C   Connections of the inflow and outflow conduits to the pump are made. The pump is de-aired, and mechanical pumping is begun as the patient is weaned off cardiopulmonary bypass. The direction of flow into the pump is depicted as if through an aortic valve. Blood is pumped out of the device by movement of a pusher plate which directs flow through the outflow conduit to the ascending aorta. The course of the transcutaneous electrical drive line, which will exit in the right lower quadrant, is shown in stippling. Drains (not shown) are liberally placed and the incisions are closed.

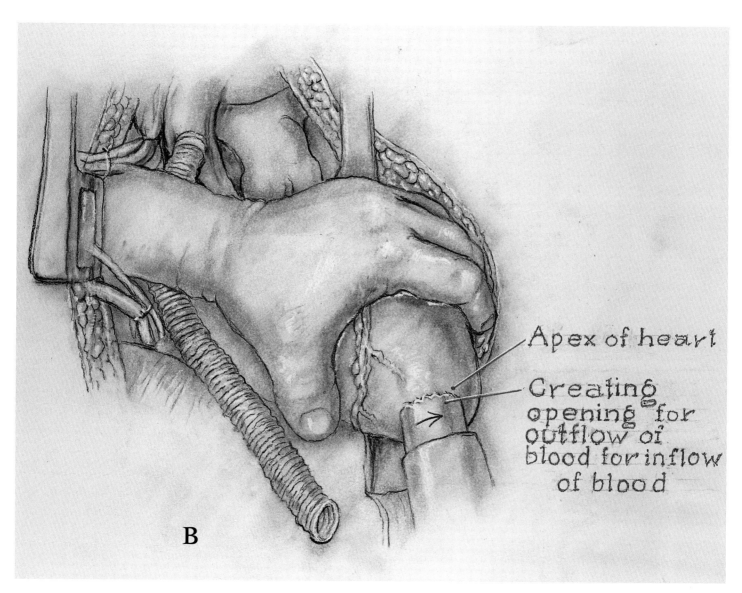

Apex of heart

Creating opening for outflow of blood for inflow of blood

B

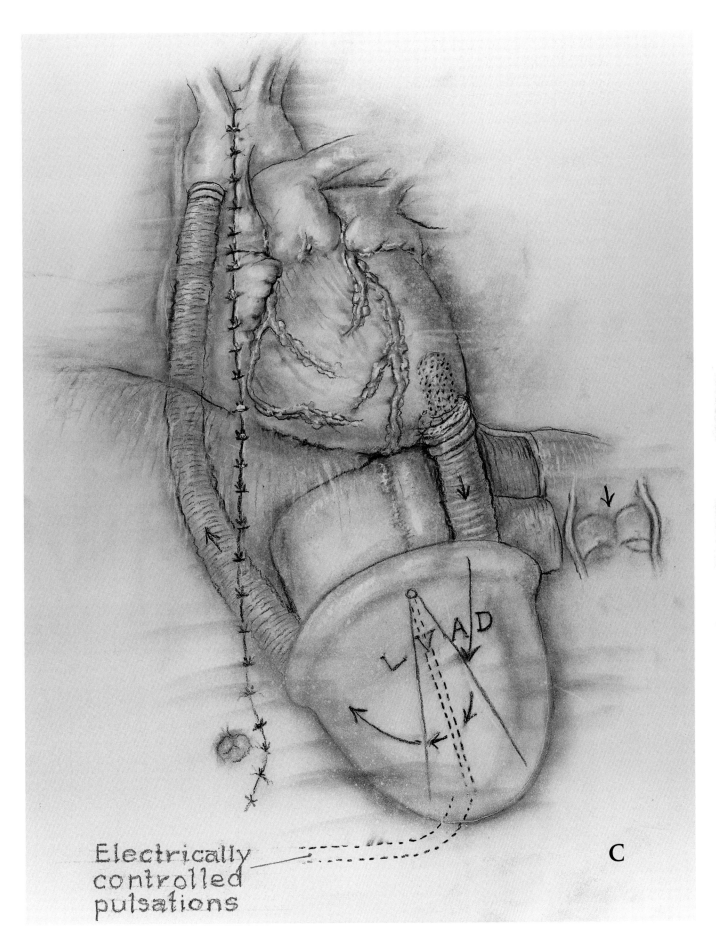

Electrically
controlled
pulsations

C

Chapter 6

Cardiac Transplantation

William A. Baumgartner, M.D.

Introduction

It has been over three decades since the first successful cardiac transplantation procedure was performed. During this period, primary advances have been made in immunosuppressive regimens, treatment of acute rejection, and reduction in the incidence of certain viral illnesses. The surgical procedure, as originally described by Drs. Lower and Shumway, is primarily used today with or without an atrial modification. Considerable experience has been gained with the standard Shumway technique, especially in the area of postoperative hemodynamics, long-term physiology, and dysrhythmias. The bi-caval anastomotic modification appears to offer some advantage in ameliorating postoperative dysrhythmias and the need for permanent pacemakers. This chapter addresses both the standard Shumway technique as well as the more recent bicaval modification.

With all the above advances, patients can look forward to extended survival with fewer complications than the pioneers endured during the early days of this experience. The availability of donor organs remains the major limiting factor to heart transplantation. However, with recent successes in the area of molecular biologic techniques, xenograft transplantation will eventually alleviate the organ donor shortage.

Donor Preparation. Because ischemic time is still limited to approximately 5 hours and is an independent variable for long-term survival, close coordination between recipient and donor teams is mandatory. Since the cardiectomy procedure is always associated with multiorgan procurement, cooperation, communication, and coordination are essential for the successful recovery of all organs. In the optimal situation, an anesthesiologist and/or nurse anesthetist accompanies the donor to the operating room and maintains vital signs during the procedure.

A-B Preparation for Cardiectomy

Following thorough prepping and sterile draping, a midline sternotomy incision is made and continued in the midline to the pubis. Visual and palpatory inspection of the heart is most important and should be performed immediately upon opening the pericardium. Special attention should be given to any palpable thrills in the area of the left atrium, aorta, and pulmonary artery. In addition, the heart should be thoroughly examined for contusions. The figure delineates the specific areas of incision. Complete dissection of the aorta and pulmonary artery superior to the level of the arch and bifurcation, respectively, should be performed. The superior vena cava (SVC) is dissected superiorly to the origin of the azygos vein and then is surrounded by two ligatures. Incomplete dissection of the superior vena cava will result in insufficient length, resulting in the ligature ties rolling off the divided ends. Proximally, this could potentially result in damage to the sinoatrial node during subsequent suture repair. The operative field becomes obscured with blood if the tie comes off the distal end of the SVC.

If separate superior vena cava and inferior vena cava recipient anastomoses are contemplated, the SVC should be dissected to the level of the innominate vein and no ligatures are used. The inferior vena cava is dissected free from the pericardial reflection to give extra length and is surrounded with umbilical tape. The aorta is then surrounded with umbilical tape, which then completes the dissection.

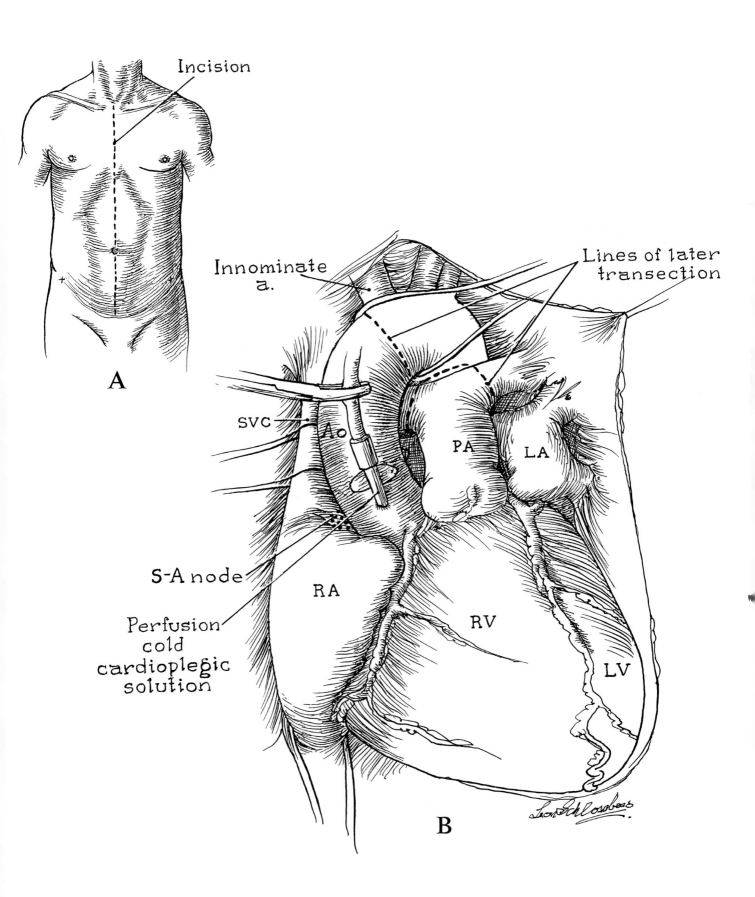

Incision

A

Innominate a.

Lines of later transection

SVC

Ao

PA

LA

S-A node

RA

RV

LV

Perfusion cold cardioplegic solution

B

C   Initiation of Organ-Protectant Solutions

Following complete dissection of the abdominal organs, heparin is administered intravenously at a dose of 300 U/kg. As hypotension occurs, both the ascending and descending aortae are simultaneously clamped at the level of the innominate and celiac arteries, respectively. We use a standard crystalloid cardioplegia solution (5% dextrose and water [D5W]) containing potassium chloride, 25 mEq/L; sodium bicarbonate, 25 mEq/L; and mannitol, 12.5 gm/L). All solutions are infused at a temperature of 2–4° C.

When hypotension has occurred, the superior vena cava is doubly ligated or stapled, and divided. The inferior vena cava is transected on the pericardial side of the diaphragm to permit egress of cardioplegic solution. With the volume-depleted heart still contracting, an aortic cross-clamp is applied and the cardioplegic solution is administered via a 14-gauge angiocatheter at a pressure of 150 mm Hg using a blood-pump pressure bag. It is important to place the angiocath as close to the cross-clamp as possible. This will allow the puncture site to be excluded when the donor aorta is trimmed. Concomitant with the administration of cardioplegia, the heart is topically cooled with cold saline.

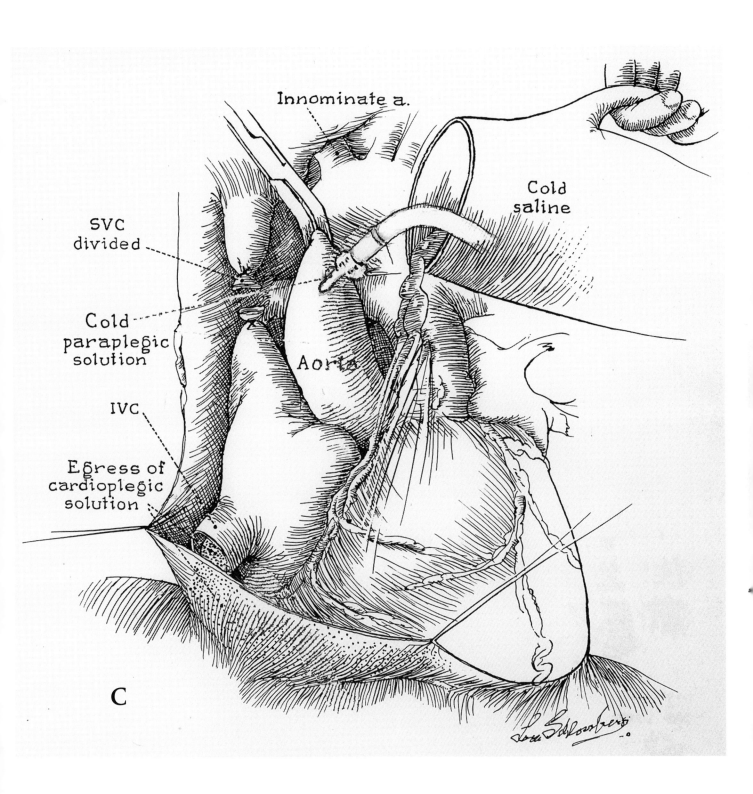

Innominate a.

Cold
saline

SVC
divided

Cold
paraplegic
solution

Aorta

IVC

Egress of
cardioplegic
solution

C

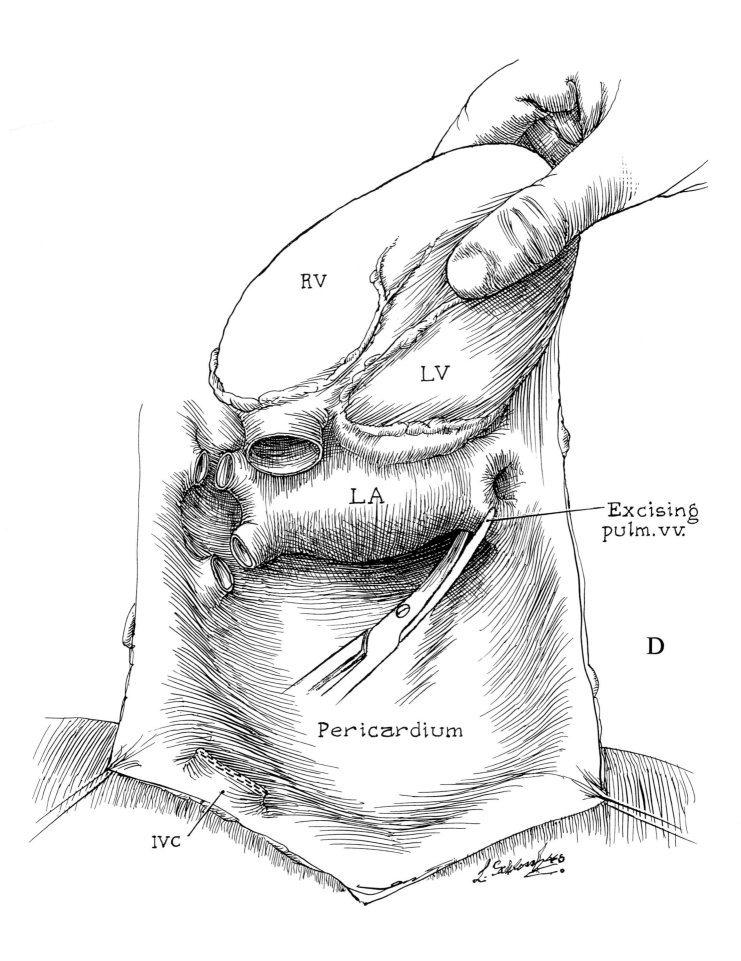

RV

LV

LA

Excising
pulm. vv.

D

Pericardium

IVC

D–E Completion of the Cardiectomy

Following arrest of the heart and division of the superior and inferior vena cavae, the heart is elevated from the pericardium and the pulmonary veins are divided individually at the level of their pericardial reflections. The pulmonary arteries are then divided beyond their bifurcation and the aorta is divided at the level of the innominate artery following removal of the aortic cross-clamp to allow additional length if needed.

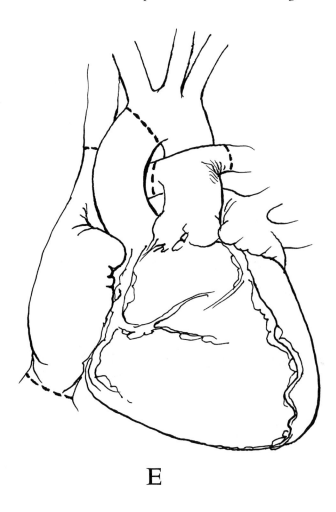

E

F–I Preparation of the Heart for Transplantation

The heart is further cooled by rinsing it in cold saline on the back table. It is then placed in two sterile bowel bags with a saline interface and subsequently placed in an air-tight container also filled with cold saline. This is placed in another sterile bowel bag, after which it is placed in a standard ice cooler for transportation.

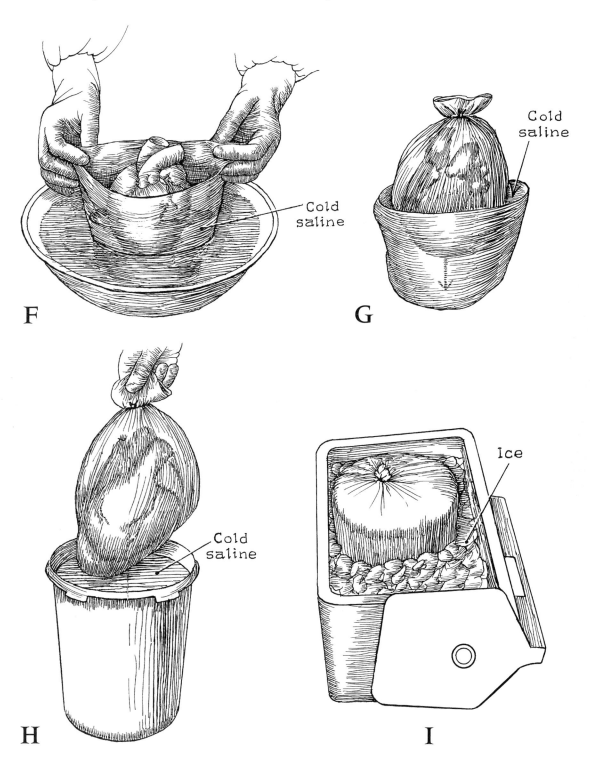

J–K Donor Heart Preparation

Preparation of the donor heart can be performed immediately following cardiectomy or when the heart is removed from the cooler at the time of implantation. We prefer the latter in order to cool the heart as rapidly as possible. The heart is then trimmed on the back table while the recipient cardiectomy is being completed. The left atrium is opened by connecting the pulmonary veins as illustrated. This provides the maximum amount of left atrial tissue, which is often needed to approximate the size of the recipient left atrium. Although the heart is not necessarily grounded, the electrocautery can be used to completely separate and dissect the aorta from the pulmonary artery. The atrial septum is checked for a patent foramen ovale, which is oversewn if present.

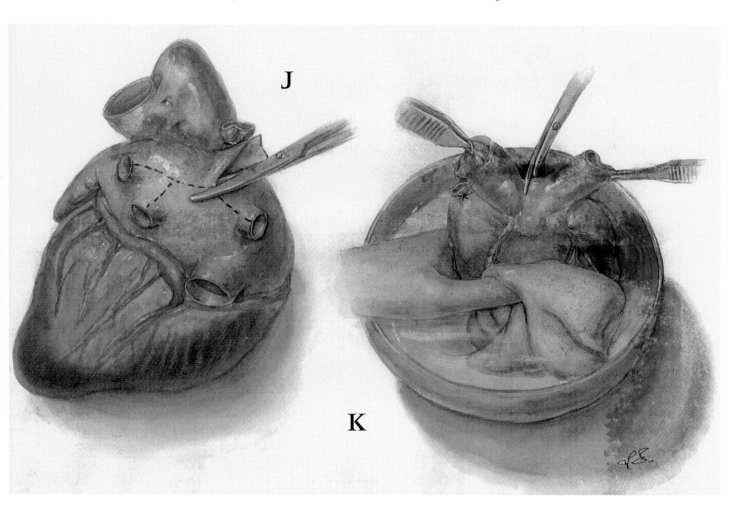

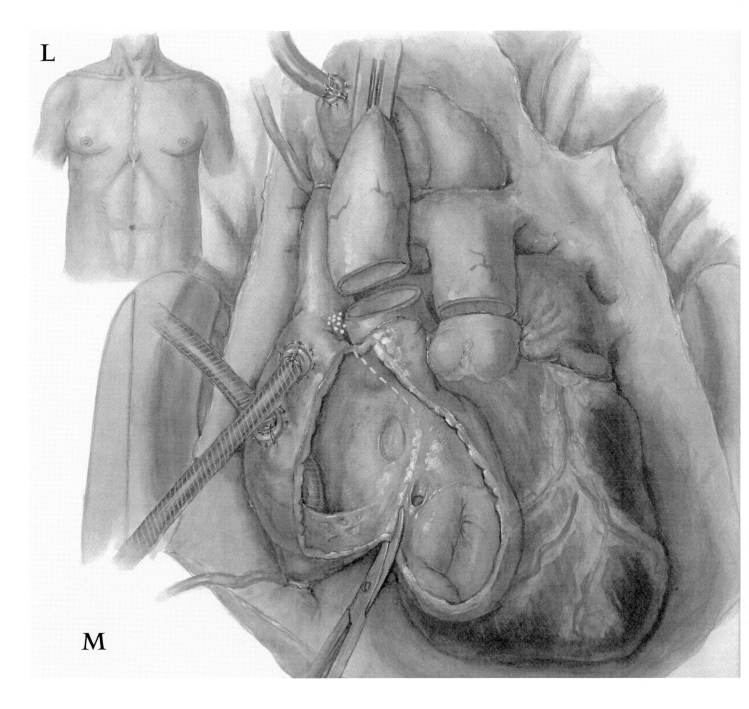

L–M Recipient Cardiectomy

The recipient operation is similar to other open-heart procedures involving a median sternotomy incision. In general, both inguinal areas are thoroughly prepped and draped. This is especially important if the patient has had a previous heart operation. Cannulation is performed centrally in the majority of cases. A 22F arterial cannula is placed as distally as possible in the ascending aorta. A 32F cannula is placed through a purse-string suture in the inferolateral portion of the right atrium and directed into the inferior vena cava. The superior vena cava can be cannulated either directly with a right-angled cannula (24–28F) or through a purse string placed in the lateral wall of the atrium at the junction of the SVC and right atrium. If biatrial anastomoses are planned, separate SVC and IVC are cannulated. The classic recipient cardiectomy operation involves complete mobilization and division of the aorta from the pulmonary artery. Both vessels are then divided at the level of the commissures of the semilunar valves. If the aortic valve is being preserved for potential allograft use, the incision in the aorta is made distal to the commissures to prevent injury. This figure depicts the great vessels divided, with the division of the atria at the level of their atrioventricular grooves posterior to the atrial appendages.

N   Left Atrial Anastomosis

Implantation of the graft begins with the left atrial anastomosis. The initial suture, a 54-inch, 3–0 monofilament nylon, is placed through the recipient atrium at the point of the excised left atrial appendage. The second arm of the suture is then placed through the donor left atrium at the base of the left atrial appendage. The heart is then lowered into the pericardium, where a previously placed cold sponge provides some insulation of the heart from the posterior mediastinum. Continuous pericardial lavage with cold saline can often be initiated at this time to maintain myocardial hypothermia. With the patient placed in modest reversed Trendelenburg and the table tilted to the patient's left, the left ventricle can often be surrounded by cold saline while the posterior suture line is made. On occasion this saline obscures the left atrial suture line, and continuous lavage cannot be instituted until this posterior anastomosis is completed.

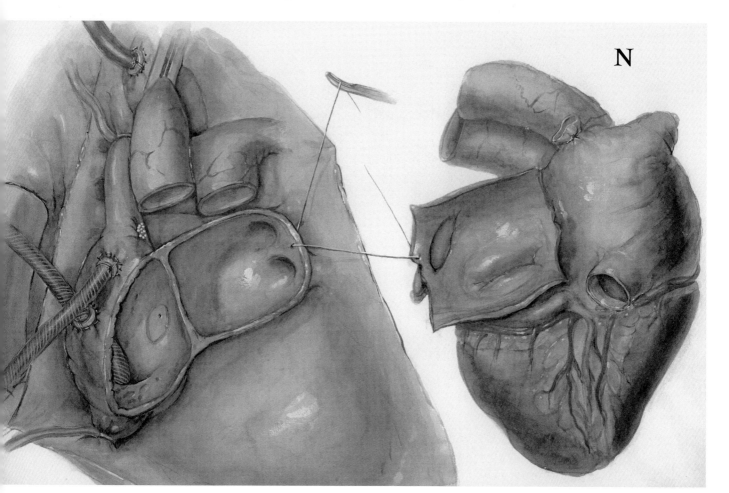

N

O–Q Use of a Left Atrial Vent

A 14-gauge vent can often be placed through the recipient right pulmonary vein and directed into the left atrium. It can also be placed in the left atrium through the donor left atrial appendage. Alternatively, we have begun placing it directly into the left atrium during the anastomosis.

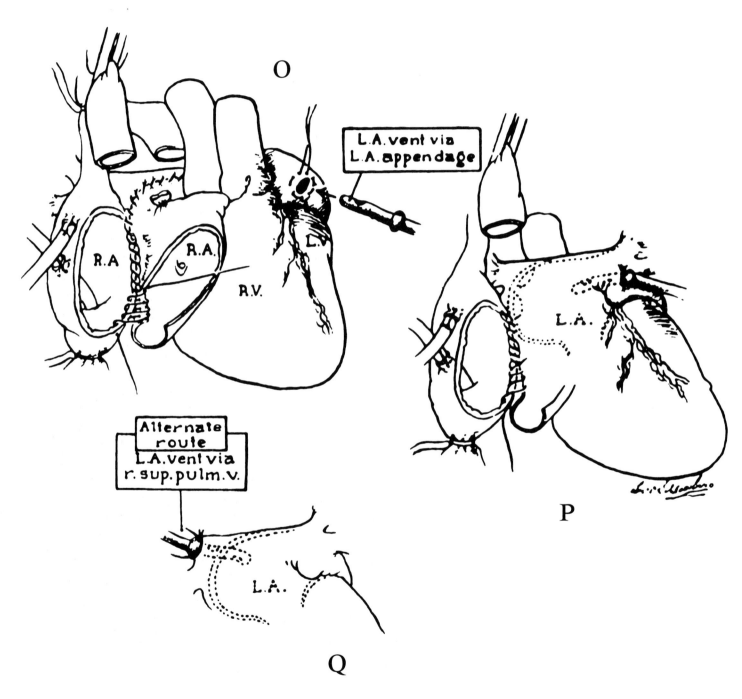

R   Completion of the Left Atrial Suture Line

Following completion of the posterior suture line, the second arm of the suture is brought anteriorly to close the left atrium at the level of the septum. The instillation of carbon dioxide gas is begun at this time. Prior to closure of the left atrium, saline is used to fill the left atrium, and generous ventilation of the lungs is employed to evacuate as much air as possible.

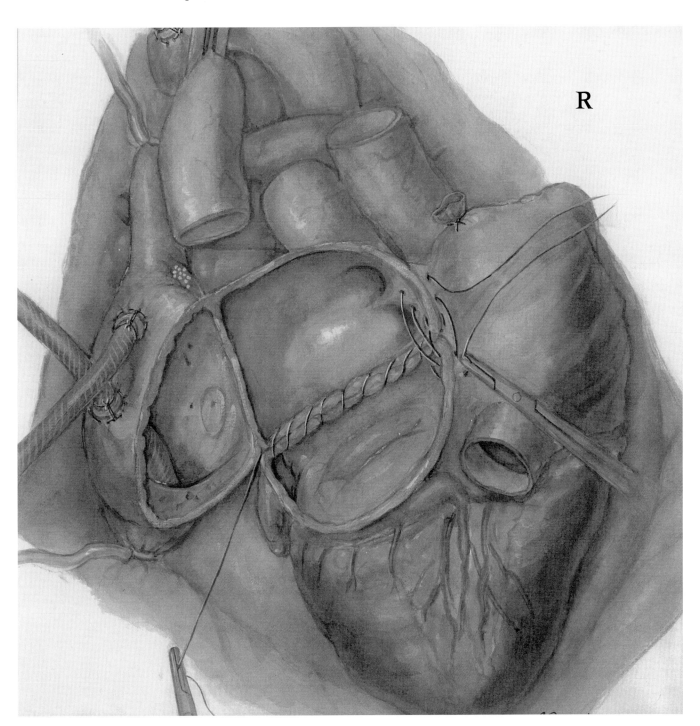

R

S   Right Atrial Anastomosis

The right atrial connection can be made in several ways. This figure shows the classic Shumway approach in which a right atrial incision is extended from the inferior vena cava upward in a curvilinear fashion into the base of the right atrial appendage. Cabrol and associates described a modification of this incision by dividing the right atrium posteriorly from the inferior vena cava to the superior vena cava. Both techniques provide protection to the sinus node. The latter technique is especially helpful when the donor right atrium is small in comparison with the recipient atrium. Also, this modification of the original technique seems to be associated with fewer dysrhythmias and increased maintenance of sinus rhythm.

The right atrial anastomosis, as depicted here, is begun at the lower end of the interatrial septum using a second 54-inch, 3–0 monofilament nylon suture. One limb of the suture is advanced inferiorly around the orifice of the inferior vena cava in an inverting manner until the suture is brought anteriorly.

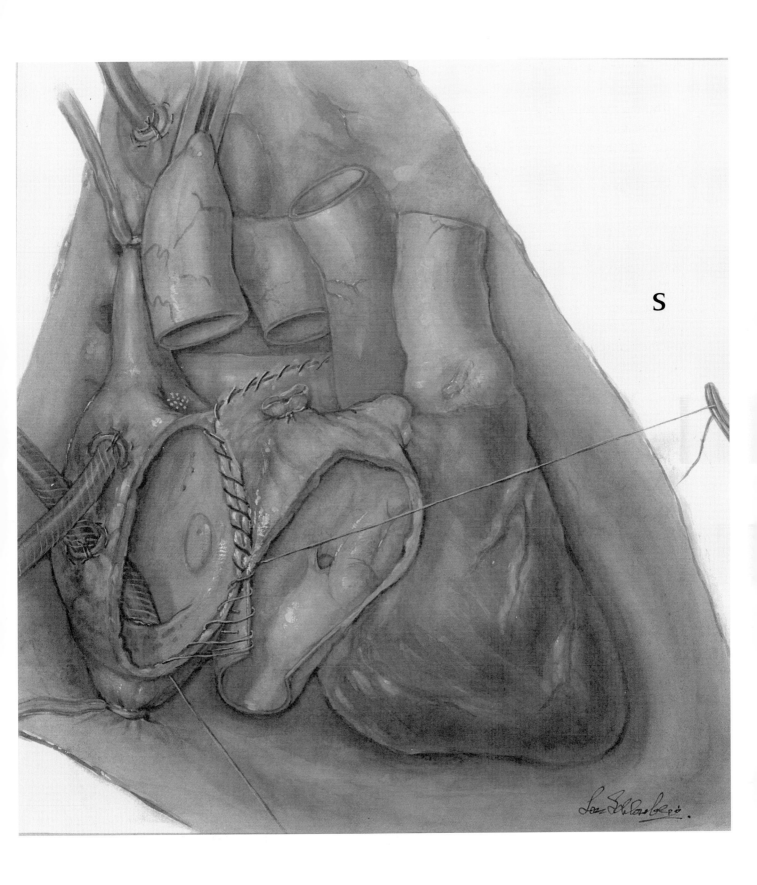

S

T Completion of the Right Atrial Anastomosis

In the standard technique, the right atrial anastomosis is completed by taking the second limb of suture and carrying it along the interatrial septum to the superior margin of the right atrium and then anteriorly where it joins the first limb. Prior to closure of the atrium, saline is used to displace as much air as possible.

T

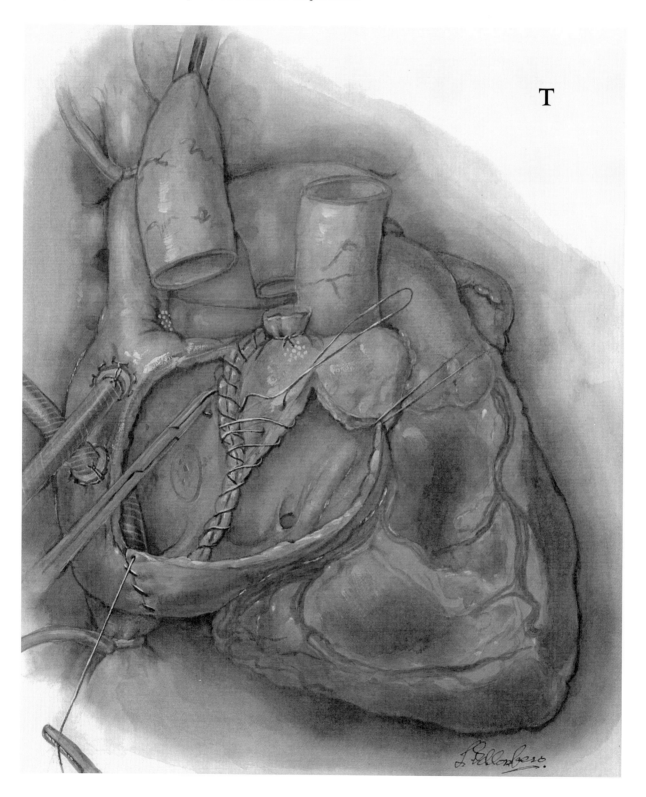

U Bicaval Technique

This figure depicts the recent atrial modification technique advocated by a number of centers. Bicaval anastomoses are completed using running 4–0 prolene suture. This technique necessitates direct cannulation of both the inferior vena cava and the superior vena cava. Small cuffs of right atrial tissue can also be used. The superior vena caval anastomosis should be performed with small bites to guard against stricture, which has been recently reported. When contemplating this technique, the donor cardiectomy should include a complete dissection of both the inferior and superior vena cavae.

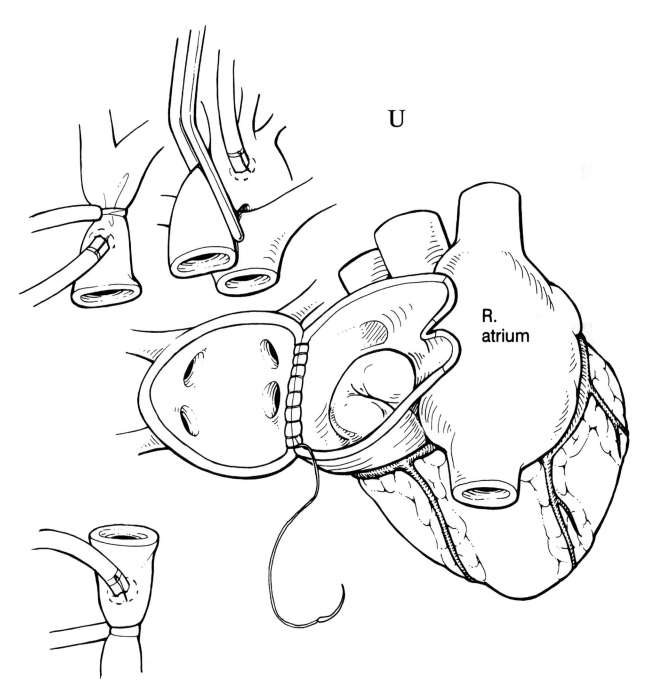

U

R. atrium

V   Pulmonary Artery Anastomosis

The pulmonary artery anastomosis is performed with a running 4–0 monofilament nylon suture, sewing the back wall from the inside and completing the anterior aspect from the outside. We usually start systemic rewarming upon completion of the pulmonary artery anastomosis.

We also release one or both of the caval snares to allow circulation of blood through the heart to initiate displacement of air during the aortic anastomosis. The pulmonary

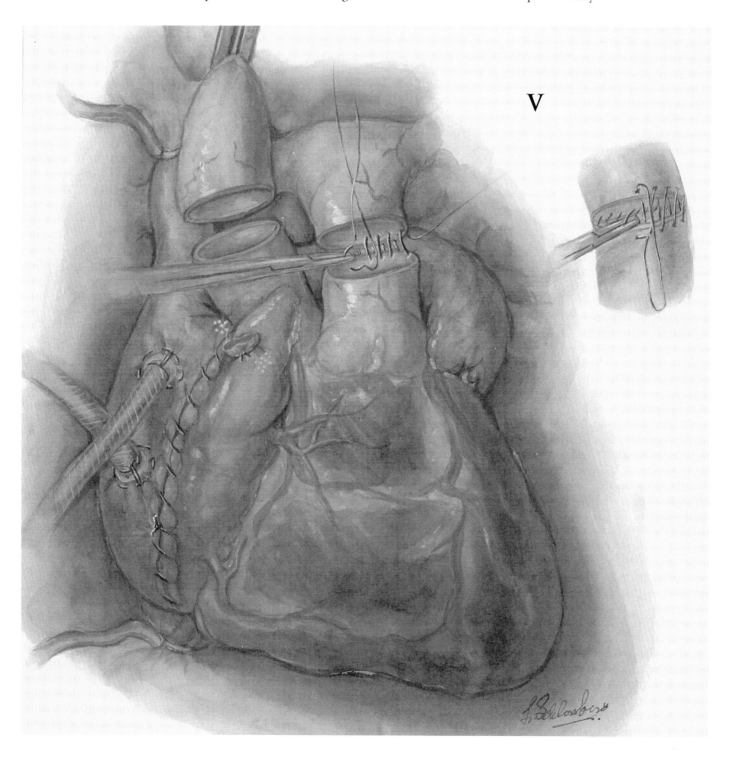

V

artery anastomosis is performed prior to the aortic anastomosis to facilitate the ease of the procedure. This method adds only 5–10 minutes to the ischemic time but provides a bloodless field to perform the anastomosis. Often, this anastomosis is performed after trimming a significant amount of both donor and recipient pulmonary artery to prevent kinking of the pulmonary artery following reperfusion.

W   Aortic Anastomosis

The aortic anastomosis is completed in a similar manner to the pulmonary artery anastomosis. The posterior wall is sutured from the inside. If there is a discrepancy in size, it is not made up on the posterior suture line. It can almost always be made up anteriorly. Prior to closure of the aortic anastomosis, vigorous attempts at air displacement are carried out.

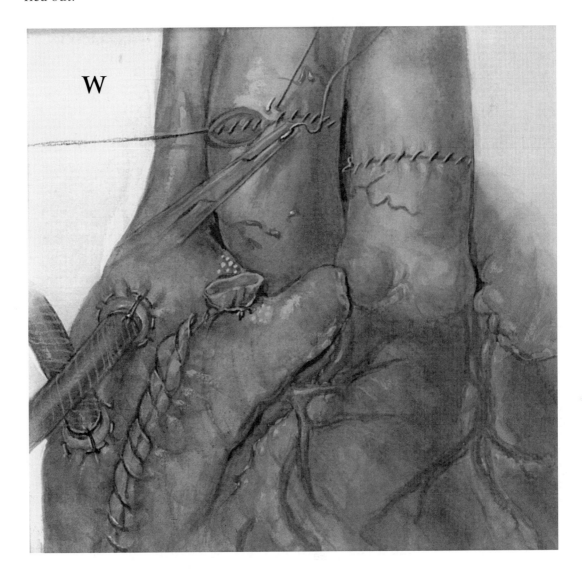

X Completion of the Transplant Procedure With Atrial Pacing Wires in Place

Once the aortic anastomosis has been completed, the patient is placed in deep Trendelenburg position, 200 mg of lidocaine is infused into the bypass circuit, and air is aspirated from the ascending aorta as the cross-clamp is released. The heart spontaneously defibrillates in approximately 50% of patients. The remaining hearts require electrical defibrillation.

While the heart is resuscitated on cardiopulmonary bypass, the suture lines are inspected. In particular, the posterior left atrial and right atrial suture lines are checked, since these are somewhat difficult to visualize after weaning from cardiopulmonary bypass. Atrial and ventricular pacing wires are then placed.

Technical Pitfalls

The displacement of air following this procedure can result in air emboli to the right coronary artery or the CNS. The former can lead to right ventricular dysfunction, which will eventually resolve following an additional period of cardiopulmonary bypass. However, in the face of pulmonary hypertension, this can be a serious problem. In an effort to reduce the amount of air in the heart, we fill the left atrium with saline and ventilate the lungs prior to closure of the left atrial suture line. In addition, we perform the pulmonary artery anastomosis prior to the aortic anastomosis in order to allow circulation of blood through the heart and through the pulmonary veins during the aortic anastomosis. The final de-airing is performed prior to closure of the aortic anastomosis. Recently we have initiated the instillation of CO_2 into the pericardial well commencing with the left atrial anastomosis. This has significantly reduced the amount of air in the heart. Transesophageal echo is often used in this procedure to assess right and left ventricular contractility following separation from cardiopulmonary bypass. It can also help to identify the degree of air remaining in the heart.

It should be emphasized again that the pulmonary artery anastomosis should be carried out without redundant tissue to avoid kinking. Conversely, the aortic anastomosis should have a certain amount of redundancy to allow easy inspection of the posterior suture line.

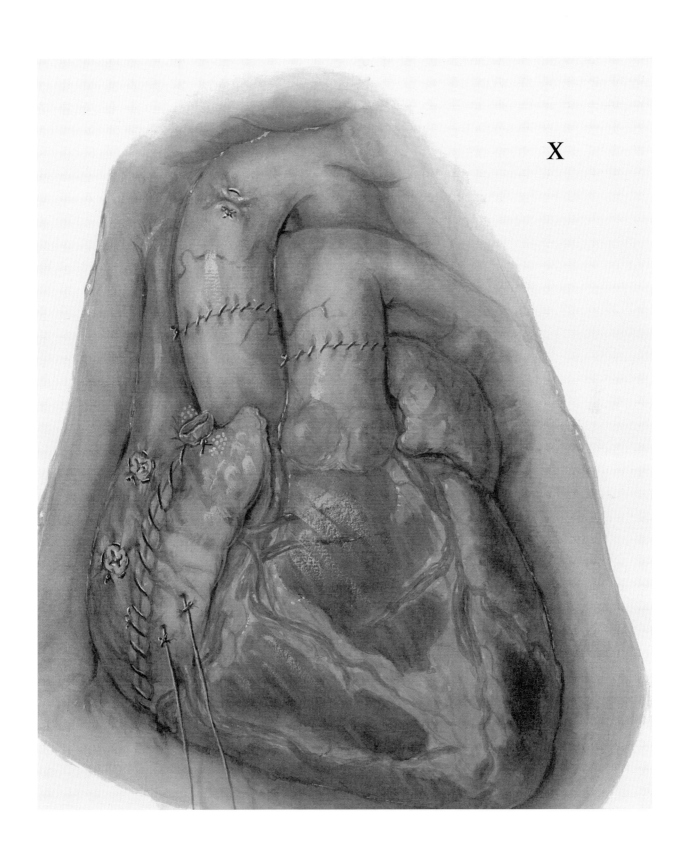

X

Chapter 7

Lung Transplantation

John Conte, M.D.

Introduction

Lung transplantation is performed for a wide variety of end-stage lung diseases. A number of surgical options exist depending on the patient's primary disease process and condition. The options include single lung transplantation, bilateral lung transplantation, and lobar transplantation. All surgical procedures share in common the need for three anastomoses: an airway anastomosis, a pulmonary arterial anastomosis, and a pulmonary venous anastomosis.

A variety of incisions can be employed to perform the transplant procedure, depending on surgeon preference. The standard approach is through a posterior lateral thoracotomy for single and lobar transplants. For bilateral lung transplantation, a sternal splitting bilateral thoracosternotomy or clamshell approach is used most commonly. Bilateral lung transplants can be performed through two separate posterior lateral thoracotomy incisions, two anterior thoracotomy incisions without sternal division in an approach similar to the clamshell incision, or much less commonly through a midline sternotomy incision.

Cardiopulmonary bypass is used in patients unable to be supported on one lung during removal of the native lung and implantation of the transplanted lung. If cardiopulmonary bypass is required during a single or bilateral lung transplant through a right thoracotomy, clamshell, or sternotomy incision, the arterial cannula is placed in the ascending aorta and the venous cannula in the right atrium. In all other approaches, the femoral artery and vein are the preferred cannulation sites.

The figures in this chapter illustrate a single left lung transplant The same steps would be repeated on the right side if bilateral lung transplantation were to be performed. The approach is through a left posterior lateral thoracotomy. The head will be oriented to the right and the feet to the left.

A   The pulmonary hilum has been exposed by opening the pericardium. The pulmonary artery and both pulmonary veins are dissected free of surrounding tissue. The inferior pulmonary ligament is divided to allow complete lung mobilization. Important structures visible are the aorta, ductus arteriosus remnant, and the phrenic and recurrent laryngeal nerves. Not visualized is the left bronchus, which lies below the pulmonary artery.

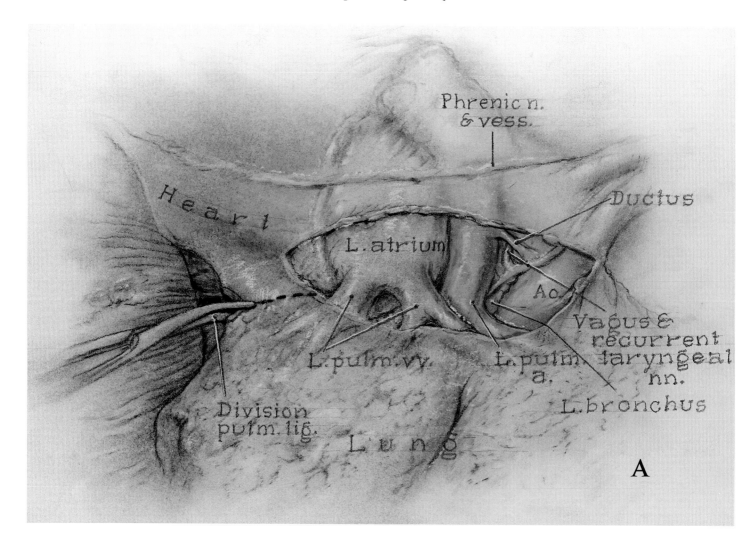

B   The inferior pulmonary vein has been divided, and the superior pulmonary vein is in the process of being divided. The pulmonary artery will be divided subsequently. Once the vascular structures are divided, the native bronchus will be exposed and divided and the native lung will be removed. The left atrial cuff, pulmonary artery, and bronchus will then be mobilized in preparation for implantation of the donor lung.

C   The donor lung has been placed in the chest and positioned for implantation. The surface will be covered with saline slush to prevent rewarming during implantation. The bronchial anastomosis has begun. The bronchial anastomosis will be constructed first, because it is the deepest and most inaccessible structure.

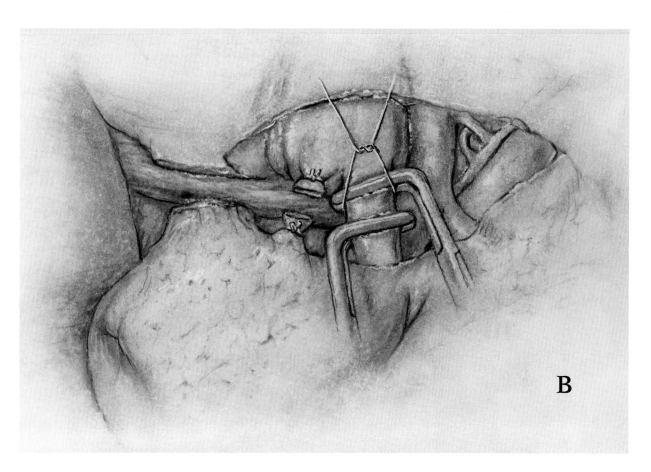

B

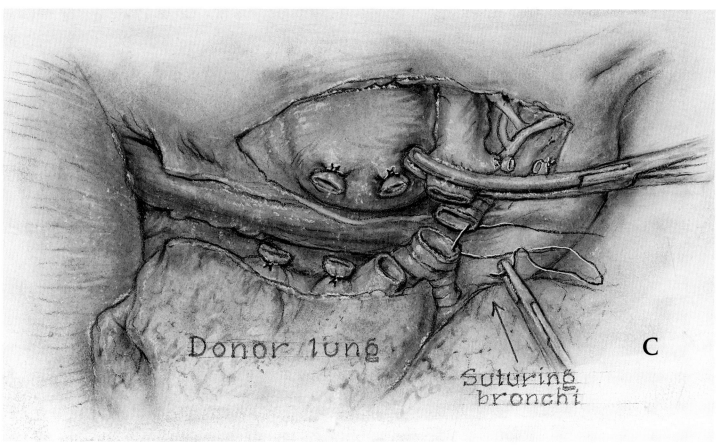

Donor lung

Suturing
bronchi

C

D   The bronchial anastomosis is shown. The two most commonly employed techniques are an end-to-end technique employing a continuous suture and an inverting technique. Sutures can be absorbable or nonabsorbable depending on surgeon preference. With the inverting technique, shown here, the membranous bronchus is sewn with a continuous suture. The cartilaginous bronchus is sewn with interrupted sutures.

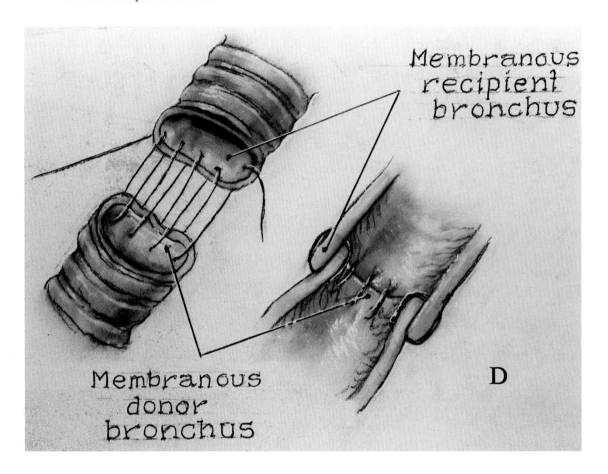

E   The cartilaginous bronchus is sewn with interrupted sutures in a figure-eight pattern. The donor bronchus is drawn into the recipient bronchus when the sutures are tightened. The sutures are tied on the external surface of the bronchus.

F   The bronchial and pulmonary artery anastomoses have been completed. The pulmonary arterial anastomosis has been constructed using an end-to-end technique with continuous polypropylene suture. A vascular clamp has been placed on the left atrium. The pulmonary veins are excised and the intervening space incised to create a cuff of left atrium for the pulmonary venous anastomosis.

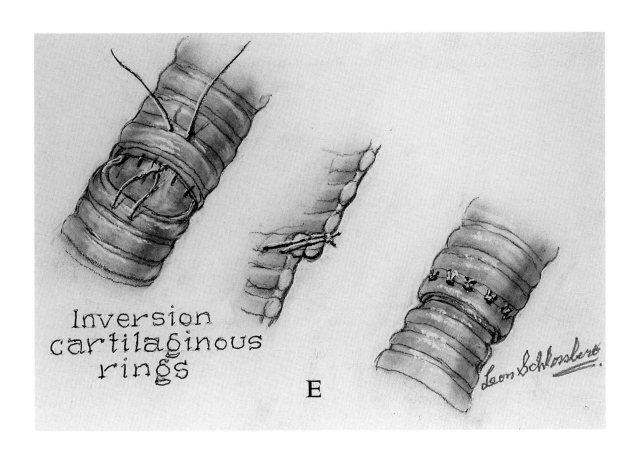

Inversion
cartilaginous
rings

E

Leon Schlossberg.

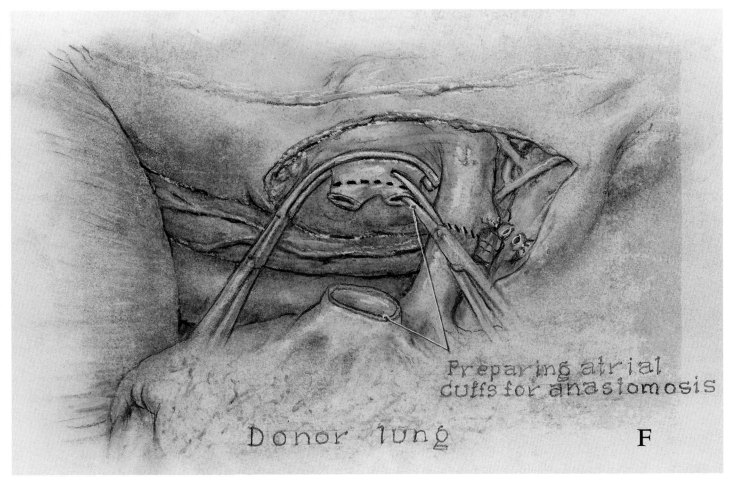

Preparing atrial
cuffs for anastomosis

Donor lung

F

G The left pulmonary venous anastomosis is under construction. The cuffs of the donor and recipient left atria are anastomosed using a continuous polypropylene suture. Retraction sutures have been placed to aid in visualization. Once this anastomosis is completed, the graft will be slowly reperfused, inflated, and de-aired. Bronchoscopy will be performed to check the bronchial anastomosis prior to closing, and a standard chest closure will be performed.

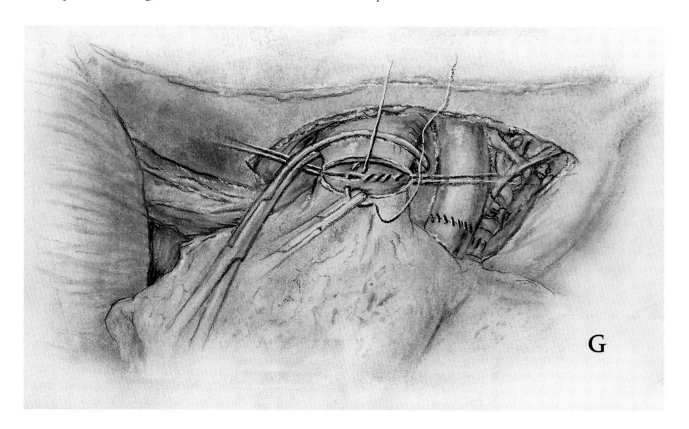

G

Chapter 8

Heart-Lung Transplantation

John V. Conte, M.D.

Introduction

Combined heart-lung transplantation is indicated for a small percentage of the population of patients with end-stage cardiopulmonary disease. It has largely been supplanted by techniques of single and bilateral lung transplantation. Patients with complex congenital heart disease with Eisenmenger's physiology whose condition cannot be repaired in the setting of a lung transplant are the most common group of patients. A second group is composed of patients with pulmonary hypertension with secondary cardiac dysfunction. Another group contains patients with end-stage lung disease and concomitant unrelated cardiac disease, such as coronary artery disease with concomitant congestive heart failure. Patients with systemic diseases affecting both the heart and lungs are another group. The operation is performed on cardiopulmonary bypass through a midline sternotomy or a bilateral thoracosternotomy or clamshell incision. The native heart and lungs are excised, leaving only the ascending aorta and right atrium intact. The alternative that is increasing in popularity is to excise the right atrium and perform anastomoses to the superior and inferior vena cavae for the systemic venous return.

A The standard approach to the recipient is through a median sternotomy, although many surgeons prefer the bilateral thoracosternotomy approach. This approach provides exposure of the heart, great vessels, and the pulmonary hilum. The anterior pericardium is opened to expose the heart, aorta, and both cavae, which are dissected and encircled with umbilical tapes.

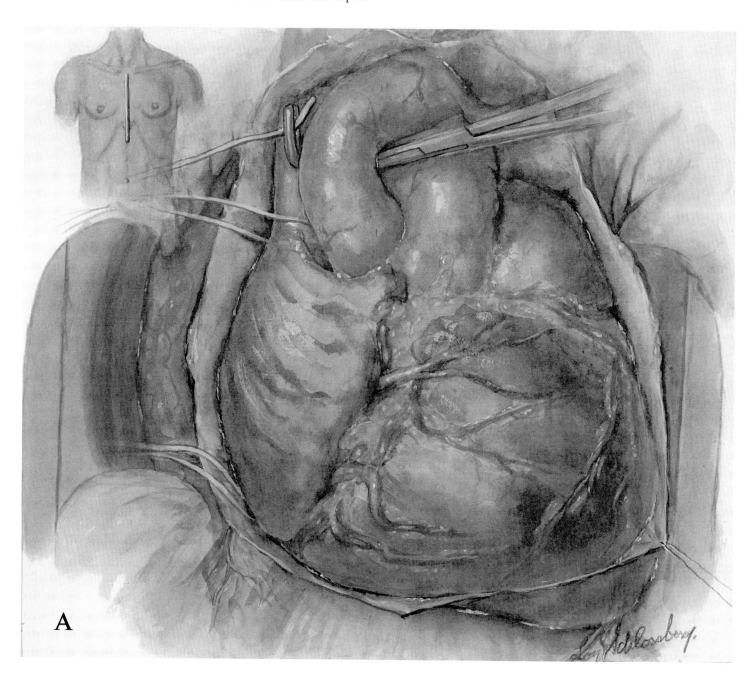

A

B The pleural spaces are entered bilaterally, and a pericardial pedicle containing the phrenic nerve is created. This is done to separate the phrenic nerve from the hilum of the lung to avoid injury during dissection of the hilar structures and to create a space for insertion of the lungs into the pleural space. The lungs may be placed into the pleural space anterior or posterior to the phrenic pedicle.

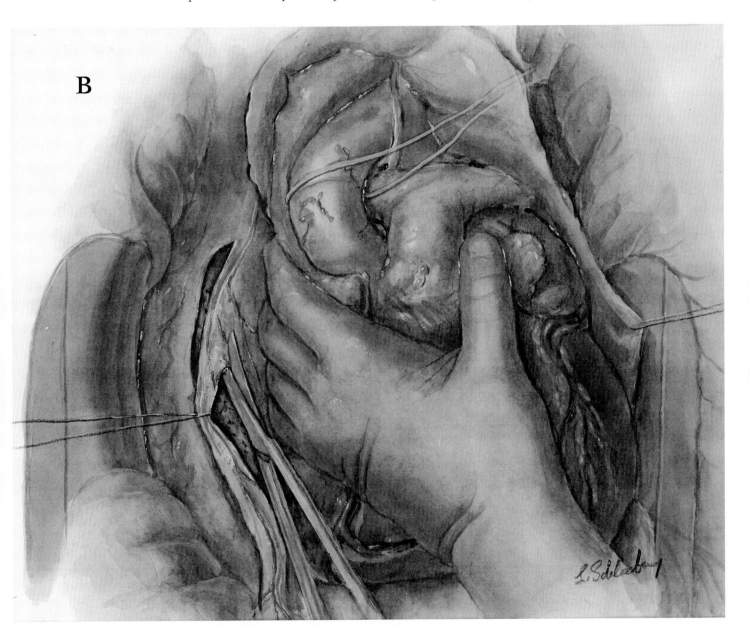

C The patient is cannulated for cardiopulmonary bypass with an arterial cannula placed in the high ascending aorta and venous cannulae placed in the superior and inferior vena cava. Once the patient is placed on cardiopulmonary bypass, systemic cooling is begun. The aorta is cross-clamped, caval snares are tightened, and the native heart is excised. The cardiectomy is performed in a fashion analogous to heart transplantation, leaving adequate lengths of aorta and right atrium for subsequent anastomoses. Unlike cardiac transplantation, left atrial and pulmonary artery anastomoses are not constructed, and these structures are removed.

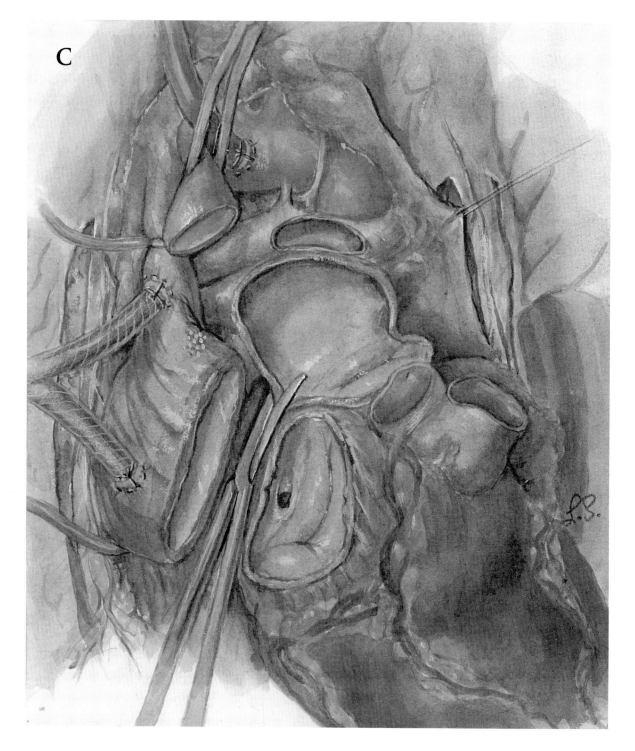

D Using gentle retraction on the phrenic pedicle, the left hilar structures are exposed and divided. The left bronchus is stapled proximal to the line of transection to prevent soilage of the pleural space. The remainder of the pleural dissection is now completed and the lung removed. Meticulous hemostasis of the hilar structures is achieved using the electrocautery.

D

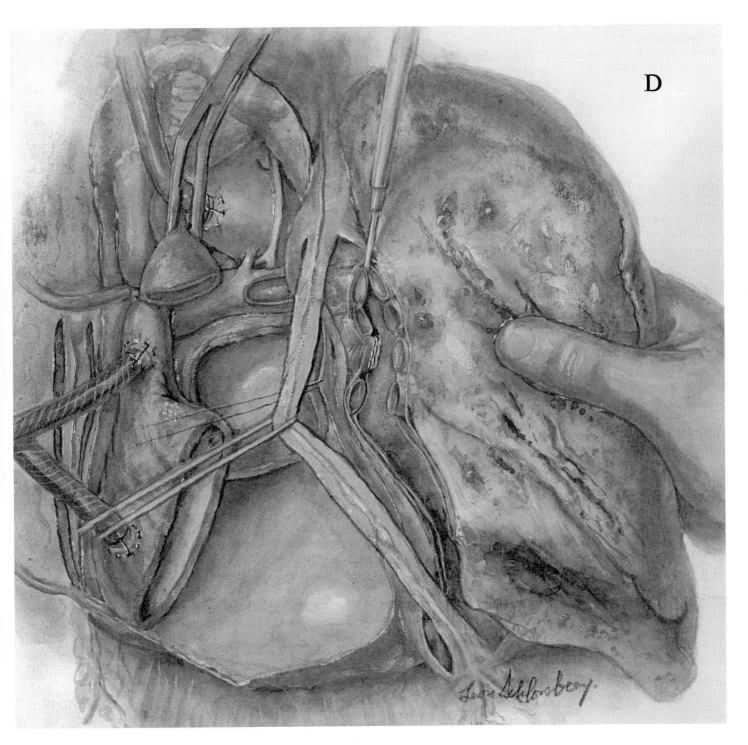

E The right pneumonectomy is performed in a similar manner. Excellent exposure of the posterior mediastinum is obtained. Hemostasis is achieved, with particular attention given to the cut edges of the pericardium, the right atrial remnant, and the mediastinal lymphatics.

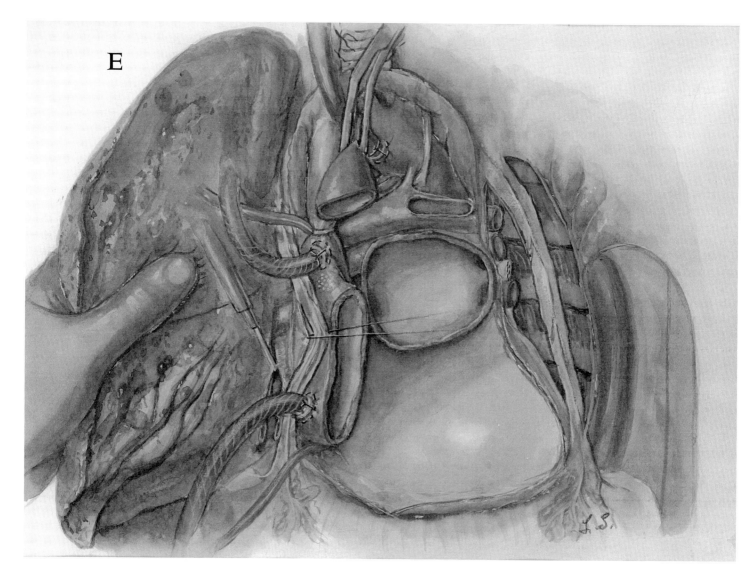

F Lungs may be placed into the pleural space anterior or posterior to the phrenic pedicle or using the alternative method shown here. A large pleural passage is developed by excising the pulmonary artery and veins as they exit the pericardium and enlarging the space by incising the pericardium cephalad and caudad. This places the donor pulmonary artery and veins in the normal anatomic position, posterior to the superior vena cava and right atrium. The left and right bronchi are removed by grasping the stapled distal ends and dissecting toward the trachea using electrocautery. The trachea is divided one cartilaginous ring above the tracheal bifurcation.

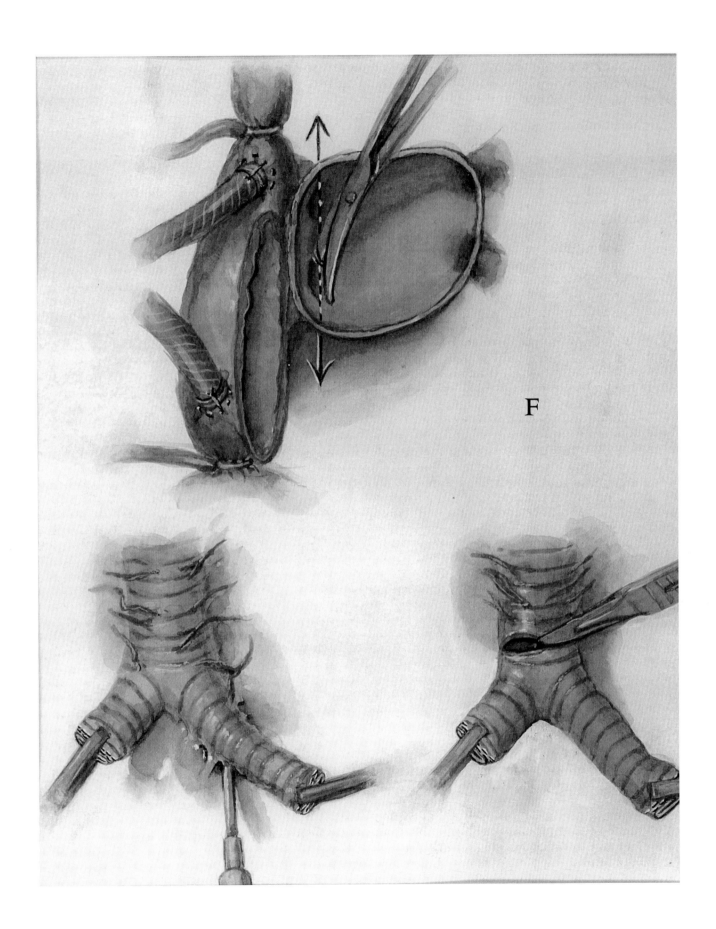

F

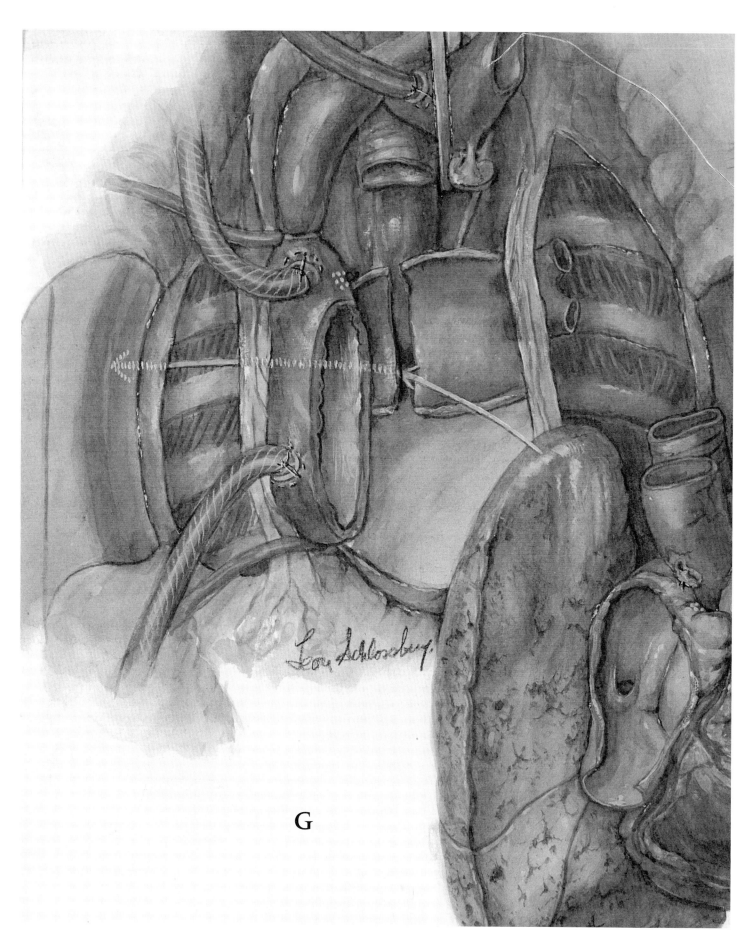

G

G The implantation begins with placing the heart-lung block into the chest. The lungs are passed into the pleural space through the spaces created. The tracheal anastomosis is constructed using a continuous polypropylene suture beginning with the posterior membranous portion.

H The tracheal anastomosis is the first anastomosis performed. Completion of the anterior surface of the tracheal anastomosis is shown. During the implantation, the donor heart and lung are kept cold by topical irrigation with cold saline or with saline slush.

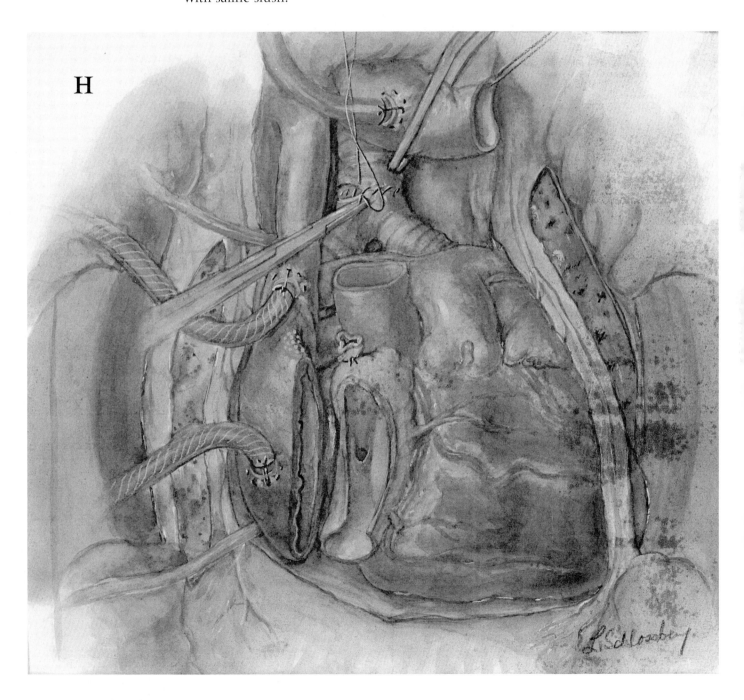

H

I   The right atrial anastomosis is constructing next using a continuous polypropylene suture technique. The donor superior vena cava has been ligated and the right atrium is opened in a manner analogous to that for cardiac transplantation, using a standard atrial cuff anastomotic technique. Alternatively, a bicaval anastomotic technique may be used.

I

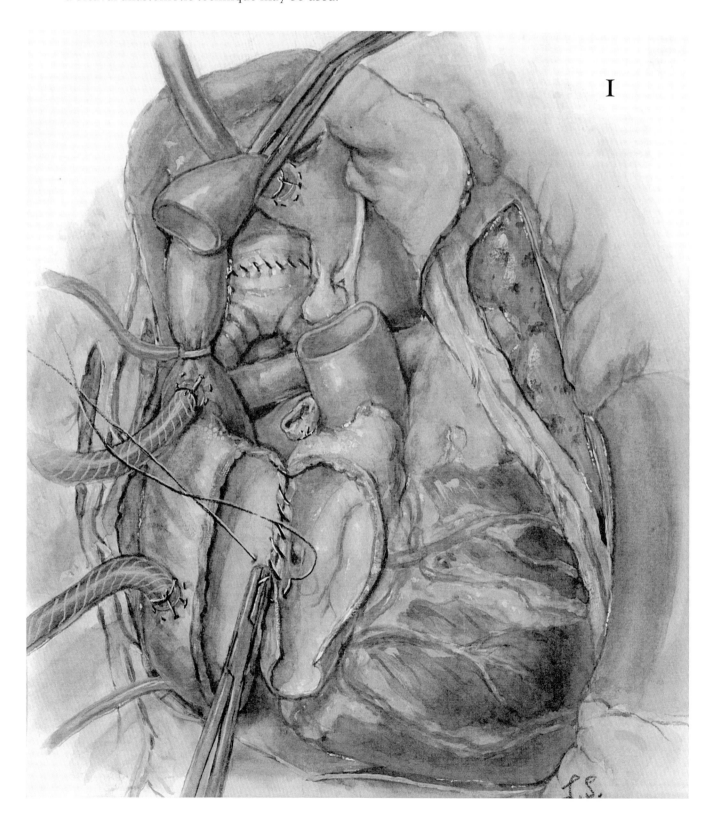

J The operation has been completed. The aortic anastomosis is constructed third, using a continuous polypropylene suture technique. The patient is rewarmed and weaned off cardiopulmonary bypass. The arterial and venous cannulae have been removed and atrial pacing wires placed. Chest drains are placed into the mediastinum and both pleural spaces.

J

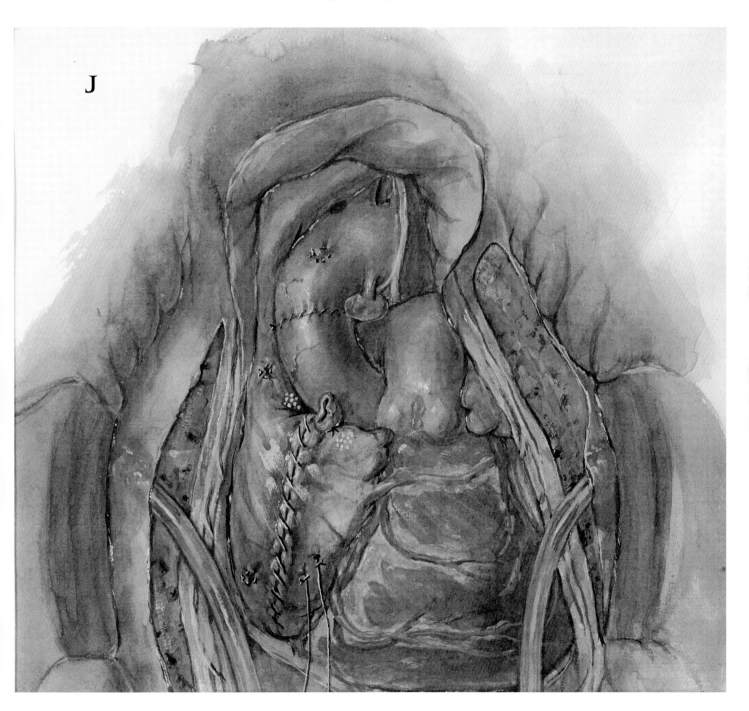

Chapter 9

Mitral Valve Approaches and Procedures

R. Scott Stuart, M.D.

Introduction

Mitral valve procedures are reasonably common in any busy surgical practice and essentially fall into the general categories of mitral valve replacement or mitral valve repair. Mitral valve replacement is now most commonly used for severe mitral stenosis and occasionally for dominant mitral regurgitation. This is secondary to rheumatic heart disease, but occasionally replacement is done for severely myxomatous valves which defy reliable repair, and for connective tissue states such as Marfan's disease. Mitral valve replacement for mitral regurgitation is sometimes performed in an older-age population or in patients with poor left ventricular function in whom the failure of the repair would not be well tolerated. Mitral valve repair itself is by far the most common procedure performed for mitral regurgitation; in some series, repair, instead of replacement, is used in up to 80% of cases. The key to adequacy and longevity of mitral valve repair lies in the basic pathology of the valve and the complexity of the subsequent repair. The more severe the underlying disease and the more complex the repair, the less confident one can be about the longevity of that repair. Regardless of repair versus replacement, the absolute requirement of all mitral valve procedures is exposure. While exposure is the dominant factor for any surgical procedure, in mitral valve surgeries truly good exposure is especially critical to a successful operation. Therefore, this chapter will begin by detailing the multiple approaches available for the mitral valve and subsequently will describe the specifics of mitral replacement and mitral valve repair.

Approaches

A-B There are three basic approaches to gaining access to the mitral valve: direct incision into the left atrium, approach through the atrial septum via the right atrium, and direct approach via the dome of the left atrium. Depicted here is the direct approach into the left atrium. Prior to making the incision, I find it useful to mobilize the inferior and superior vena cava in the region of their respective confluences to the right atrium itself. This allows for extension of the left atrial incision underneath the structures if required. At this time I cut the pericardial stay sutures on the left side of the retractor. This will allow the pericardium and the heart to fall deeper into the left chest and improve the angle of visualization onto the mitral valve. The incision itself is best begun at the level of the superior pulmonary vein and is made approximately 5 to 10 mm medial to the confluence of the superior vein with the left atrium. Occasionally, thick epicardial fat may be encountered. Once in the left atrium, the incision is carried inferiorly to a position below the inferior pulmonary vein. Further extension of the incision underneath the IVC and/or SVC is performed at this time, depending upon the view of the mitral valve.

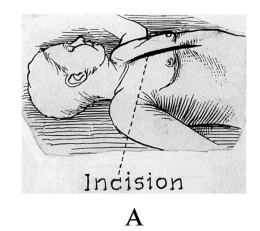

Incision

A

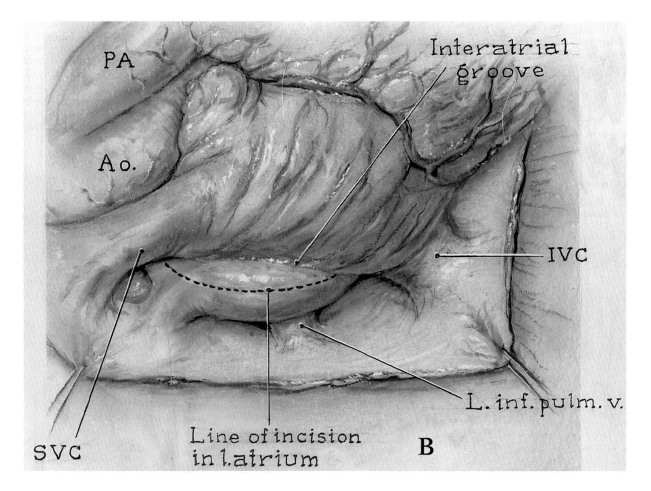

B

C–E The variation on the direct approach to the left atrium is illustrated. Waterston's groove (the groove demarcating the junction of the right and left atrium) is occasionally easily appreciated. A shallow incision is made in this region which is more medial than the line of the standard incision depicted above. This groove may be exploited medially for several millimeters, which will allow a better angle of approach to the mitral valve. This incision also requires the mobilization of the SVC and IVC for maximum exposure.

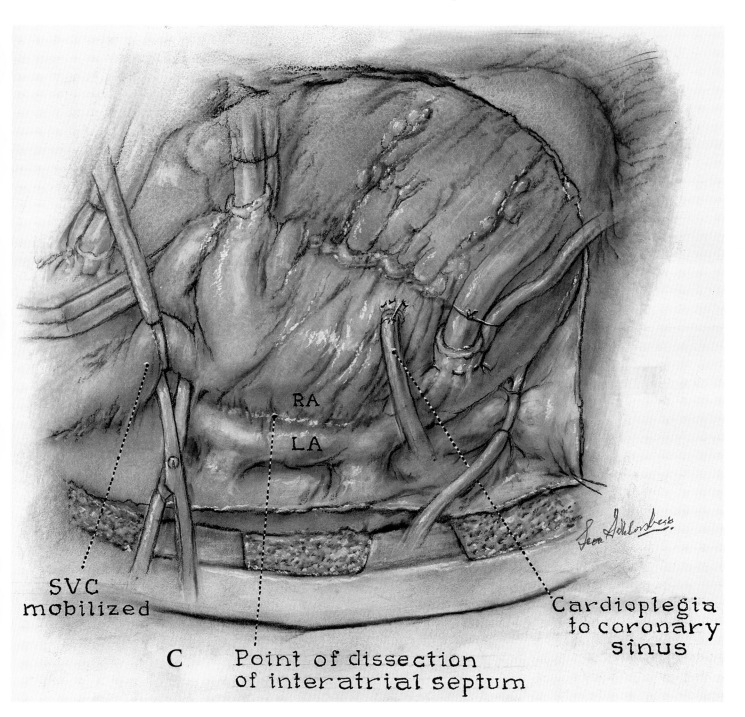

RA

LA

SVC
mobilized

C   Point of dissection
of interatrial septum

Cardioplegia
to coronary
sinus

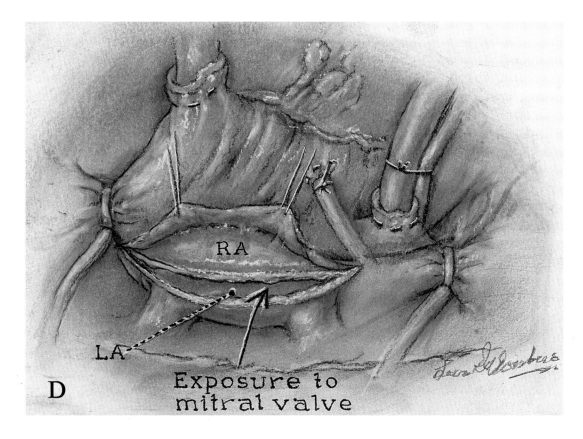

D

Exposure to
mitral valve

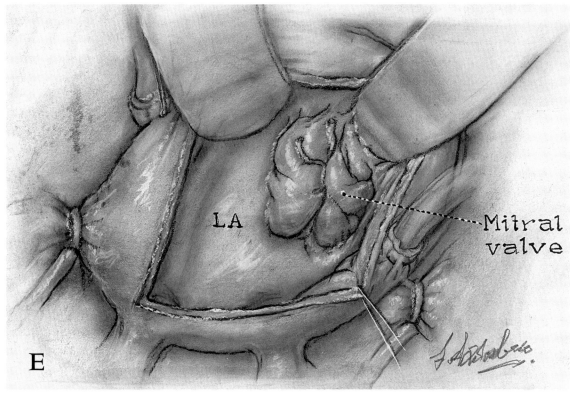

E

F The first major alternative to approaching the mitral valve involves opening the right atrium and crossing the atrial septum. Such approaches have been beneficial in that the angle of approach to the mitral valve is more acute and the view often superior to that of the traditional left atrial approach. This approach is frequently useful in a reoperative setting, where the rotation of the heart may be limited by adhesions. It is also useful in a teaching situation in that the attending surgeon (in the assistant's position at the patient's left) usually will have an excellent view of the entire mitral valve and thus will feel much more secure in allowing the fellow to proceed with the case. As with a standard approach, double venous cannulation is required. I prefer direct cannulation of the superior vena cava to allow a cleaner operating field through the right atrium. Incision into the right atrium is made after institution of cardiopulmonary bypass, administration of cardioplegia, and engaging the Rumel tourniquets. This incision may be made in a horizontal fashion, as depicted here, or in a vertical fashion extending from the point of the forceps in this illustration to just above the atrial septum in a line heading toward the superior pulmonary vein. One advantage of this incision is that a separate left superior vein vent may be inserted, which will allow for excellent venting of the lower left atrium without the cannula being within the operative field.

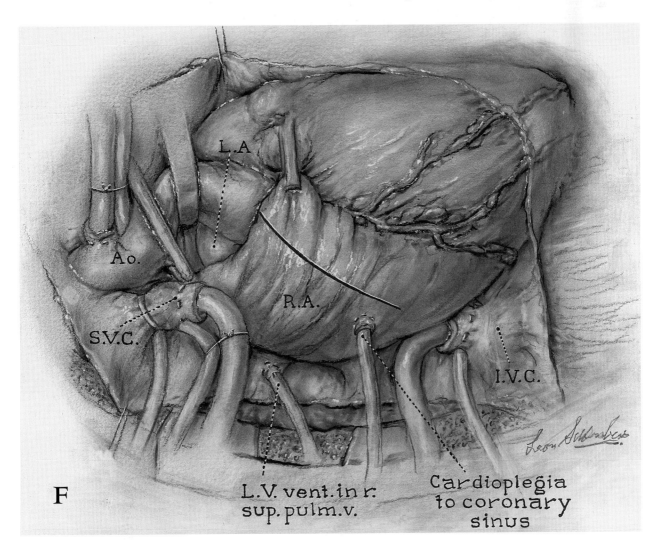

Approaches *continued*

G–H With the right atrium opened, the fossa ovale should be easily appreciated. Incision is made within the fossa and extended superiorly and inferiorly to gain better exposure of the mitral valve. The extent of this incision is kept well within the left and right atria. At this point I use two vein retractors inserted into the upper aspect of the incision to provide better visualization of the mitral valve. Occasionally, this view may be augmented with a very small malleable retractor. This limited incision is more than adequate to carry out almost any mitral procedure.

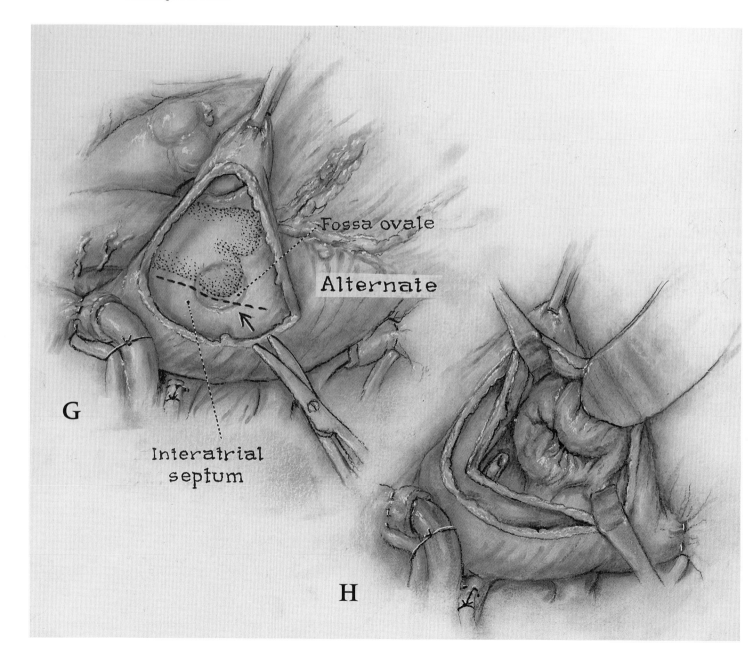

I–K If one is not satisfied with the exposure obtained with the limited incision just described, then this incision may be extended into a superior transeptal incision. The superior aspect of the septal incision is continued and thus it will cross the "northern border" of the right atrium and can be carried into the dome of the left atrium. Such an incision is extended in a stepwise fashion with frequent inspections of the access gained to the mitral valve. It is most commonly used in reoperative situations, where exposure is severely limited. If full extension of the incision onto the dome of the left atrium is required, the terminal aspect of this incision should be biased toward the left superior pulmonary vein and not toward the base of the left atrial appendage. Tissue in the region of the left atrial appendage is notoriously fragile, whereas tissue in the region of the superior pulmonary vein is of much better integrity for subsequent closure of the incision.

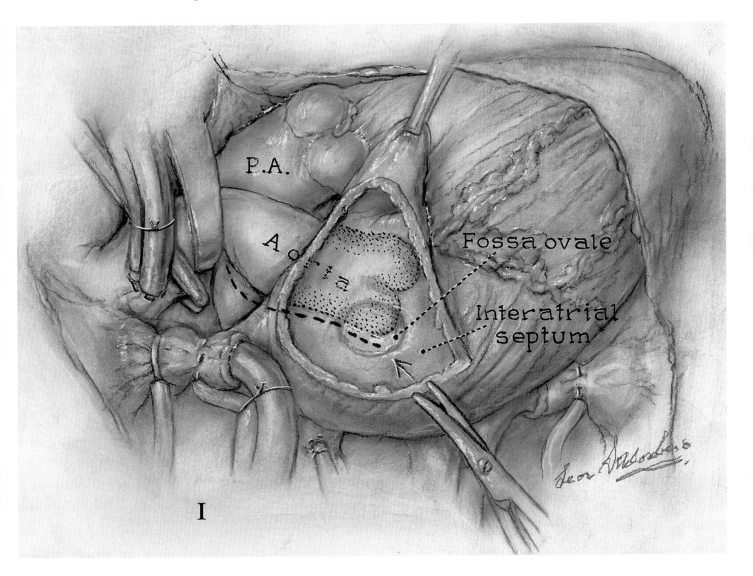

I

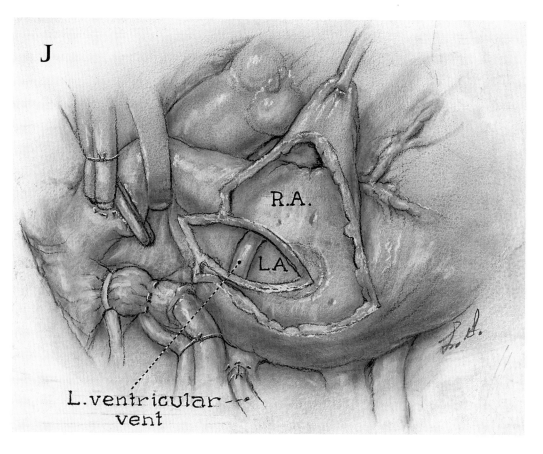

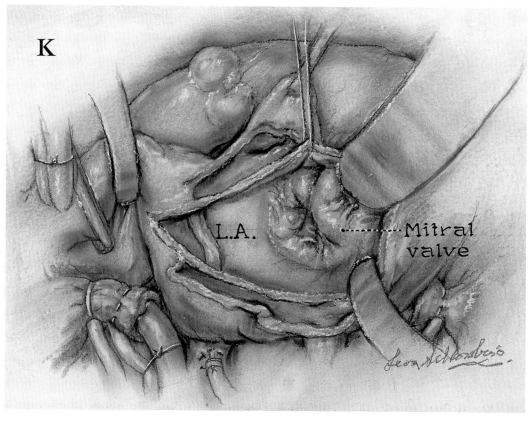

L A variation on the right atrial/septal approach is illustrated. The incision is made into the right atrium in a vertical fashion and carried down not only to, but across, the atrial septum at the region of Waterston's groove and onto the medial aspect of the superior pulmonary vein.

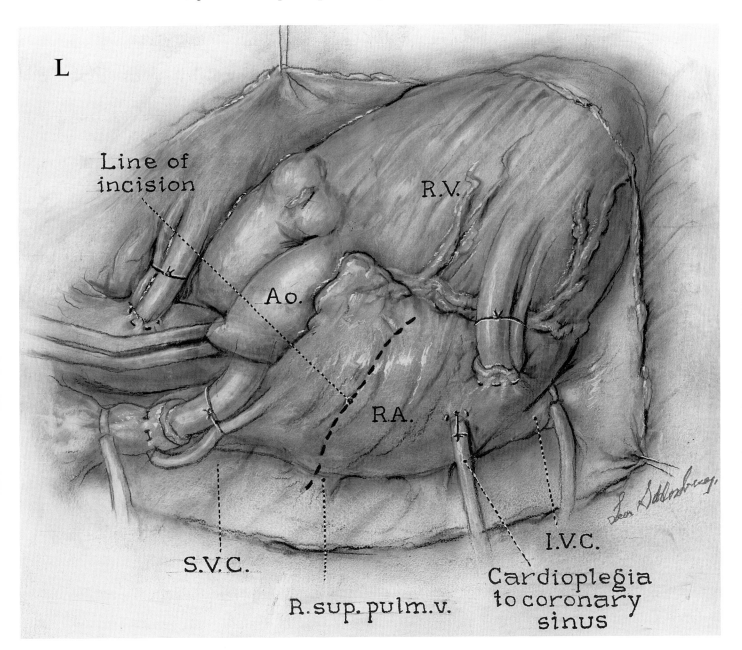

Approaches *continued*

M This original incision in Figure L is continued by dividing the septum in a line which passes through the fossa ovale. The septal incision stops at the medial aspect of the fossa to avoid inadvertent injury to the nodal apparatus in the triangle of Koch.

N When fully developed, excellent exposure of the mitral valve may be obtained. This incision, often termed a book incision due to its resemblance to opening a book, is frequently useful in reoperative situations where adhesions are quite severe and mobility of the right and left atria may be quite limited.

M

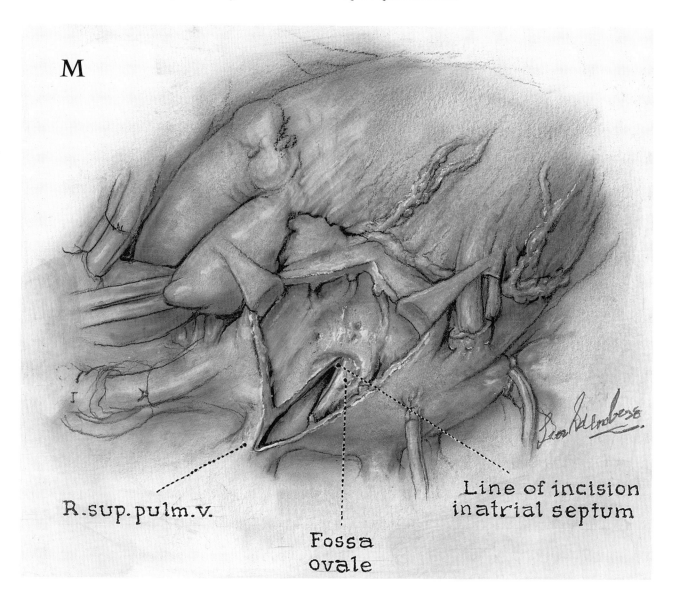

R.sup.pulm.v.

Line of incision in atrial septum

Fossa ovale

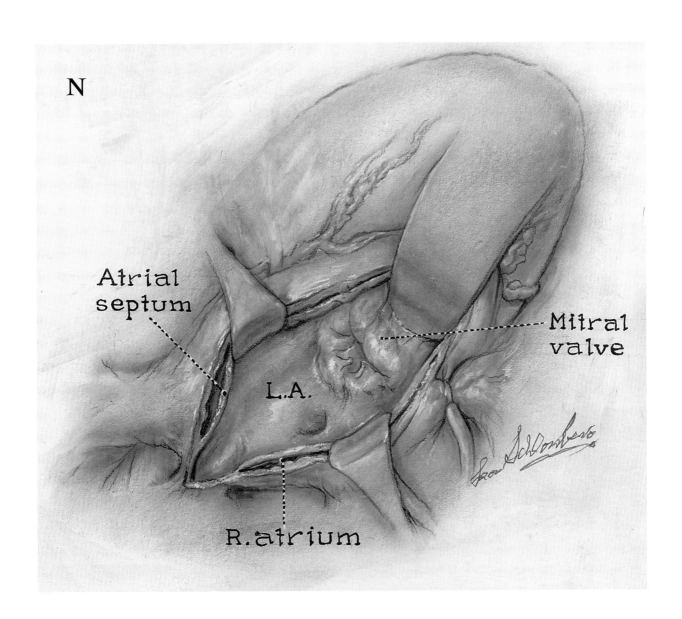

Atrial
septum

Mitral
valve

L.A.

R. atrium

Other Approaches

For the sake of completeness two other approaches, though rarely used, should be mentioned. The first is approaching the mitral valve solely through the dome of the left atrium. This can be performed in a heart with an extremely enlarged left atrium. The line of approach is in the dome of the left atrium between the aorta and superior vena cava and requires lateral retraction of each of those structures. Another use of this incision is in those patients requiring ascending aortic and or aortic root replacement.

The dome of the left atrium is easily approached after transection and removal of the diseased segment of the ascending aorta. The root is pulled anteriorly, and free access to the dome of the left atrium is acquired. Incision is made directly into the dome with a subsequent approach to the mitral valve. Again, if the incision is extended to the left lateral aspect of the atrium, the line of an incision terminates toward the left superior pulmonary vein instead of the base of the left atrial appendage. This second unusual approach is actually via a right thoracotomy with direct access gained through the left atrium. The incision itself into the left atrium is identical to that of the standard left atrial approach but is carried out through the thoracotomy. A better explanation and depiction of that approach is included in the chapter on minimally invasive procedures.

Mitral Valve Replacement

A   Mitral valve replacement is usually required in cases of moderate to severe mitral stenosis and in cases of mitral regurgitation where the abnormality of the valve and/or the subvalvular mechanism is so severe as to preclude reliable repair. With the mitral valve accurately exposed, removal is begun by first grasping the anterior leaflet with forceps or even an Allis clamp. Traction is placed downward and outward, and an incision with a number 15 blade is made at the 12:00 position, horizontally, approximately 2 to 3 mm from the annulus itself. This incision is carried around the circumference of the anterior leaflet maintaining the 2 to 3 mm distance from the annulus. This incision may be extended with a knife or scissors. With severe mitral stenosis, the subvalvular mechanism is frequently scarred and contracted, and retention of the mechanism is impossible. It is useful to employ a right-angle clamp placed around the thickened chordae to aid in their division. This improves visualization of the chordae and protects the underlying ventricular muscle. Great care must be taken when passing the right-angle clamp to avoid clamp-induced tears into the ventricle. Chordae are divided at a location just before the head of the papillary muscle. Not dividing the papillary muscle itself prevents inadvertent "buttonholing" of the ventricular wall, which can later present as a blowout from the weakness caused by such an incision. Division of the chordae to the anterior leaflet is best accomplished after detachment of the leaflet from the annulus. With the anterior leaflet removed, the posterior leaflet exposure is markedly enhanced. Removal of the posterior leaflet is accomplished in a similar fashion, usually beginning with the detachment of the leaflet from the annulus. However, the chordal structures are much more easily viewed in the absence of the anterior leaflet, and it may be that dividing the chordae should be accomplished first. The subsequent rolling of the leaflet mechanism outward into the operative field thus facilitates the final division of the leaflet from the annulus.

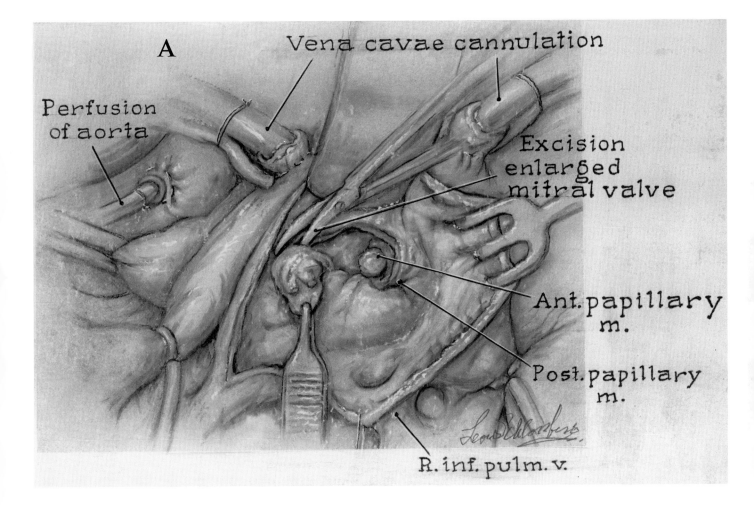

A

Vena cavae cannulation

Perfusion of aorta

Excision enlarged mitral valve

Ant. papillary m.

Post. papillary m.

R. inf. pulm. v.

Mitral Valve Replacement *continued*

B With the leaflets and subchordal mechanism fully resected, any areas of calcification in the annulus are debrided at this time. Subsequently, valve sutures are placed in the mitral annulus. We use everting mattress sutures (with or without pledgets, depending on the integrity of the annulus) when using a prosthetic valve.

An everting technique may also be used with tissue valves. However, should the tissue valve be better served by a "boiler plate" technique, then those mattress sutures are placed through the annulus in a direction from ventricle to atrium. As shown in this illustration, there are two key areas where large suture bites should be avoided.

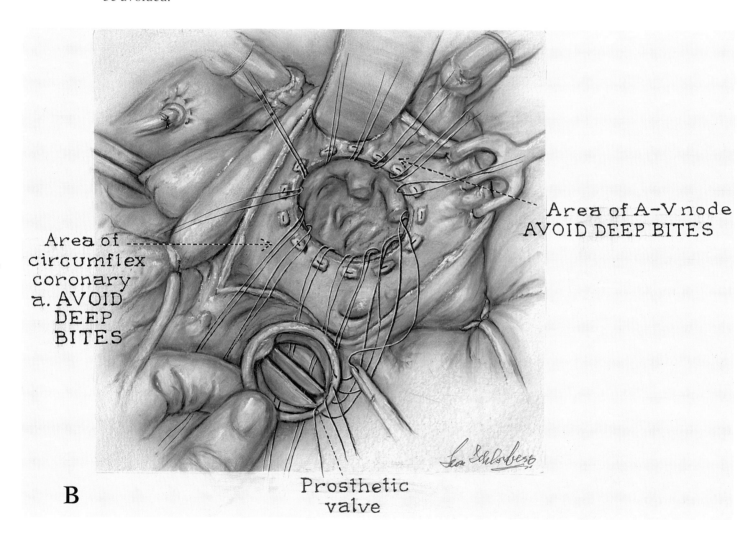

Area of circumflex coronary a. AVOID DEEP BITES

Area of A-V node AVOID DEEP BITES

B

Prosthetic valve

1. In the area contiguous with the aortic valve. Deeper bites in this region may impinge on the AV node and may also compromise subsequent functioning of the aortic valve itself. Therefore, placement of sutures in this region (from the 11:00 through 1:00 position as viewed by the surgeon) should be quite evenly spaced and no attempt made to "make up" distance in this area.

2. The other region in which to avoid deep bites is at the 4:00 through 8:00 position of the annulus. Beneath this area lies the circumflex artery and

coronary sinus, either of which may be compromised by an aggressively placed suture. After placement of the valve sutures, their individual members are passed through the sewing ring of the given prosthetic valve. Tissue valves afford a normal natural division of the sewing ring into thirds due to the natural cusp formation. Most mechanical valves now come equipped with sewing-ring markers which will divide the ring into thirds or quadrants. Should this not be available on the valve, use a sterile marking pen to divide the ring into quadrants or thirds to facilitate placement of the valve sutures.

C-D Preservation and retention of the chordae is to be desired, since clear evidence exists that subsequent ventricular function is improved if the subvalvular mechanism is retained during mitral valve replacement. This is most easily accomplished in valves in which severe mitral regurgitation is present and the valve cannot be adequately repaired. Such leaflets and their subvalvular mechanism are often pliable enough to allow "reefing" underneath the prosthetic valve. Occasionally, stenotic valves will have some chordal mechanism which can be retained. These two illustrations depict the retention of chordae. In this case, the leaflet tissue itself has been removed and only the chordae with a small remnant of tissue has been retained. Larger amounts of leaflet tissue with secondary and tertiary chordae may also be retained and are often easily reefed beneath the mitral annuli when an everting mattress suture technique is used. If significant chordal and/or leaflet material is retained, it is important that everting techniques with mechanical valves be used. Again, if tissue

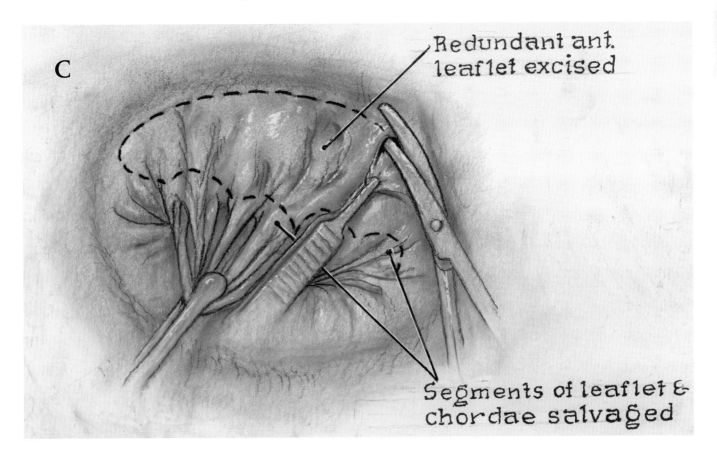

C

Redundant ant. leaflet excised

Segments of leaflet & chordae salvaged

Mitral Valve Replacement *continued*

C-D *continued*

valves are used, boiler-plate suturing technique may be employed. With this technique, it is important that the first pass of the suture catch the edge of the leaflet and gather its bulk underneath the anulus prior to passing the suture through the mitral annulus itself. Such a technique is most commonly used with bioprosthetic valves.

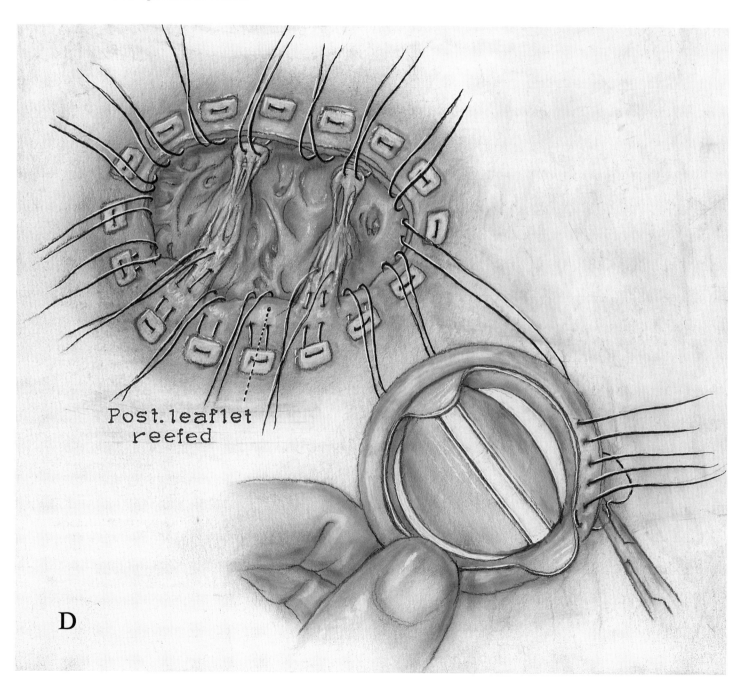

Post.leaflet reefed

D

E   After the valve sutures have been passed through the sewing ring of the prosthetic valve, traction is maintained on the ends of the suture and the valve "parachuted" down into the mitral annulus. Prior to tying the sutures, the subvalvular area is inspected. With prosthetic valves, the end of the cotton swab is applied to the leaflets (to avoid scratching the artificial surface). For bioprosthetic valves, a small dental mirror may be gently inserted through the orifice of the valve to ensure that no sutures have become looped around the valve stents. Valve sutures are tied with a minimum of six throws.

The sutures are then divided, leaving only 1 to 2 mm of "tail" above the knot. This avoids longer suture ends becoming entangled in the leaflet mechanism of mechanical valves. Prior to closure of the atrium, a small red rubber tube or Foley catheter (size 10 or 12F) may be inserted through the leaflets of a mechanical valve to minimize the trapping of air within the ventricle during subsequent de-airing procedures. After de-airing is concluded, the catheter, which has exited through the atrial closure line, is gently retracted. We recommend that bioprosthetic valves not be stented with such a device due to the high likelihood that the delicate leaflets may be torn during removal of the catheter.

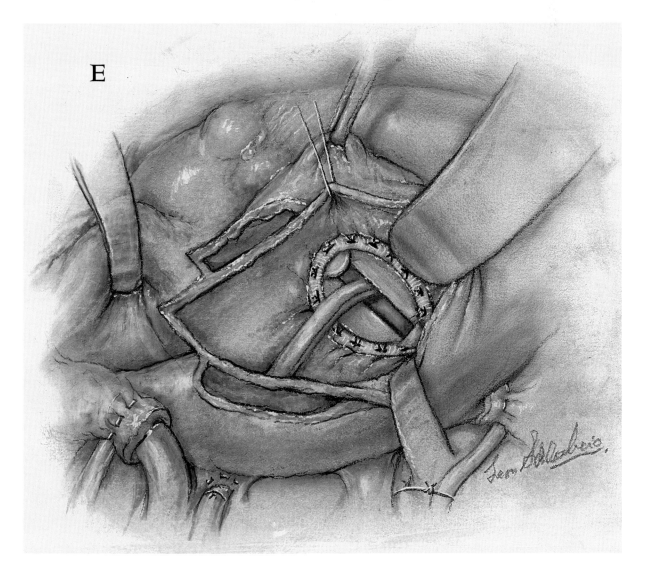

Mitral Valve Repair

Mitral valve repair is a general phrase encompassing many procedures performed upon the mitral valve, exclusive of mitral valve replacement. These procedures may range from simple commissurotomy, in the case of early rheumatic mitral stenosis, to chordal transposition with annular remodeling and neochordal construction. This segment of the chapter will discuss the dominant forms of repair from most simple to more complex.

A-B One straightforward form of mitral valve repair is mitral commissurotomy. This is most frequently indicated in early mitral stenosis when the valve is experiencing commissural fusion but still has a relatively mobile subvalvular apparatus. As depicted in the figure, the commissures are opened along their natural line by sharply dividing the fused commissures with a #15 blade. The proper line of incision may be clarified by providing retraction on the anterior and posterior mitral leaflets. The incision itself is carried to, but not into, the mitral annulus..

The figure also shows the more complex repair involved in the release of the thickened chordae and even delamination of some of the leaflet thickening. As shown, shallow incisions are made along the position of the dotted line in the figure. The vertical incisions will often be sufficient to increase mobility of the chordae themselves. The leaflets, however, will often require a true stripping or delamination of the thickened scar tissue. Occasionally, the chordae will have to be shaved to increase their mobility. This form of repair for mitral stenosis is actually quite rarely required and, frankly, the results may be somewhat disappointing. One may be able to obtain fairly good leaflet and chordal mobility in the operating room only to find, several weeks or months later, that the patient has "re-stiffened" that valve and will ultimately require a redo operation for mitral valve replacement. Therefore, such chordal shaving and leaflet delamination should be restricted to those patients who are suffering from relatively mild to moderate mitral stenosis. In fact, the vast majority of such patients will probably be best served by mitral valve replacement.

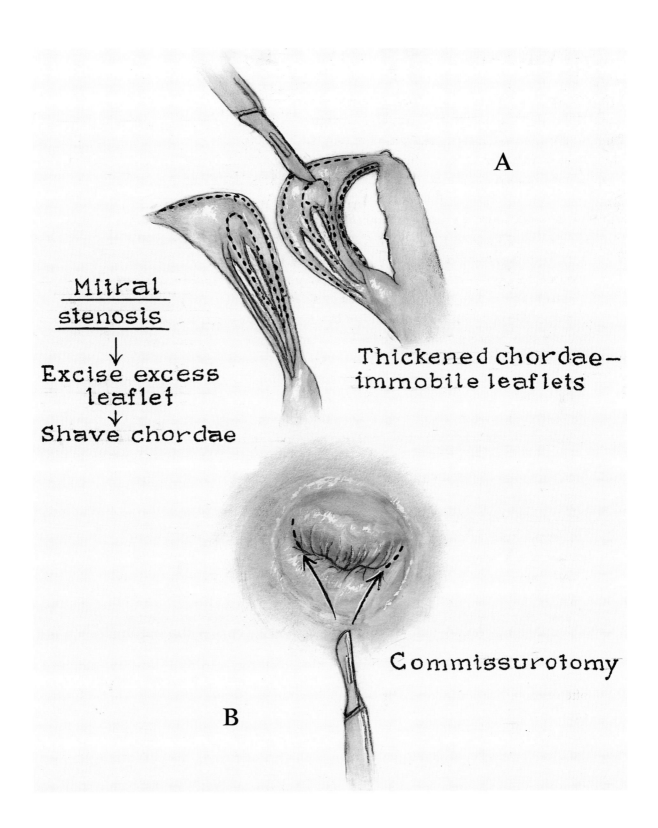

A

Mitral stenosis
↓
Excise excess leaflet
↓
Shave chordae

Thickened chordae-immobile leaflets

Commissurotomy

B

Mitral Valve Repair *continued*

C   The next simplest form of mitral repair is that depicted in figure C. It is the Reed, or Kay, annuloplasty. It is most easily applied in cases of mitral regurgitation where there is little true organic mitral disease and the regurgitation is commonly secondary to other valve lesions such as aortic stenosis. The repair is effective only in those patients with virtually no annular calcifications, since the annulus must be mobile enough to withstand the plication as depicted in the figure. The annuloplasty itself is carried out with a 3-0 or 4-0 braided suture, although prolene is equally satisfactory. The annuloplasty begins by placement of a pledgetted horizontal mattress suture in the area of the trigone. The sutures pass through the annulus, beneath the anterior and posterior leaflets, and exit through the posterior leaflet annulus in a location approximately one fourth to one fifth along the length of the posterior mitral annulus. Free pledgets are placed on the end of the horizontal mattress sutures, and the effective annular circumference is reduced. The distinct advantage of this annuloplasty is that it is simply and quickly performed and usually gives good, but not excellent, reduction in the given amount of regurgitation.

Reed Annuloplasty

Decreasing size of annulus opening

C

D   Many patients who experience moderate to severe mitral regurgitation are found to have basically normal-appearing valves when directly viewed by the surgeon. Frequently these are patients who have either severe non-mitral cardiac disease (such as aortic stenosis or insufficiency which has engendered secondary mitral regurgitation) but, most commonly, they are patients with congestive heart failure often from a dilated cardiomyopathy. In these patients, a large mitral annulus causes the regurgitation due to lack of proper coaptation by the anterior and posterior leaflets. Valvular competence is restored by reducing the size of the mitral annulus. To select the proper size ring, one can measure the valve in either of two fashions. The most common form of measurement involves grasping the anterior leaflet, providing downward traction to place the anterior leaflet on a stretch, and subsequently matching the size of that leaflet to the appropriate ring sizer. The subsequent repair will ensure that an adequate reduction in annular size is obtained without too severe a degree of reduction, which would result in effective mitral stenosis. The second method of measurement involves applying the ring sizer directly to the anterior mitral annulus. Such sizers will have preformed marks on the upper and lateral corners of the sizers. These marks will correspond with the commissure or the trigone, depending on the given manufacturer. Care must be taken to ensure that the surgeon realizes which marks are meant for which location. Once a proper size ring is chose, 2-0 braided sutures (most frequently without pledgets) are placed through the mitral annulus in an everting fashion. For rings such as a Duran ring or classic Carpenter "D" ring, the annular sutures will be placed in a completely circumferential manner as depicted in figure D. After placing the sutures through the annulus, they are brought through the ring itself, the ring lowered onto the mitral annulus, and seating assured as the sutures are tied. At the completion of the procedure, the integrity of the repair may be tested by manually instilling sterile saline through the mitral valve

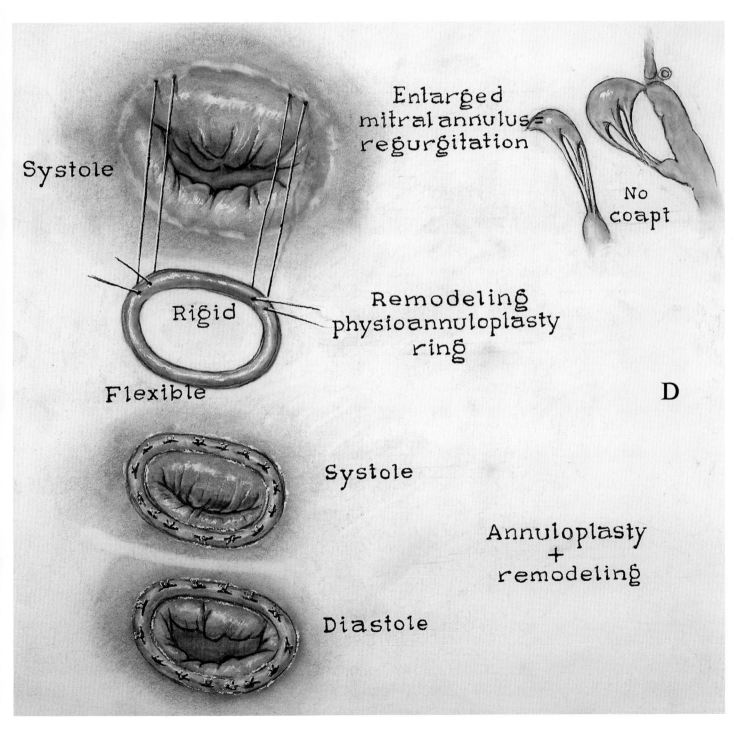

Mitral Valve Repair *continued*

D *continued*

itself. Such installation should be reasonably firm and followed by a rapid with-drawal of the tube from the mouth of the annulus. Overly forceful installation of saline into the ventricle can actually entrap and force ventricular air into the cross-clamped aortic root, which will subsequently cause that air to travel down the coronary artery after removal of the clamp. Finally, the left atrial appendage is closely inspected to ensure there is no thrombus, and the appendage may be closed from within using a purse-string suture at the base of the appendage with a 3-0 or 4-0 prolene suture. Alternatively, the appendage may be tied off externally by using a large-gauge braided tie.

E

A common cause of mitral regurgitation is chordal elongation, most frequently seen in myxomatous valves. Elongation will commonly, though not always, precede chordal rupture. It is rare that a single elongated chord will be responsible for significant mitral regurgitation. Most frequently, three or more chordae will be elongated in significant regurgitation. The traditional method of chordal shortening is depicted in figure E. It involves making a vertical cut with a #15 blade into the true center of the papillary muscle, which controls the elongated chordae. Following this, a 4-0 or 5-0 prolene suture is looped around the one or more chordae to be shortened, and the ends of that suture are subsequently brought through the base of the "V" in the papillary muscle. The chordae are tucked into that "V" and the suture subsequently tied over a free pledget. The papillary "V" is closed and reinforced with a pledgeted 5-0 prolene horizontal mattress suture. Such a technique of chordal shortening will often produce a very satisfactory repair. However, it has been our experience that such shortening will often not retain its integrity over the course of multiple years. Perhaps this is due to the fact that abnormal chordae are simply being shortened and the primary pathology within the chordae is not truly addressed. Regardless, our current preference is to

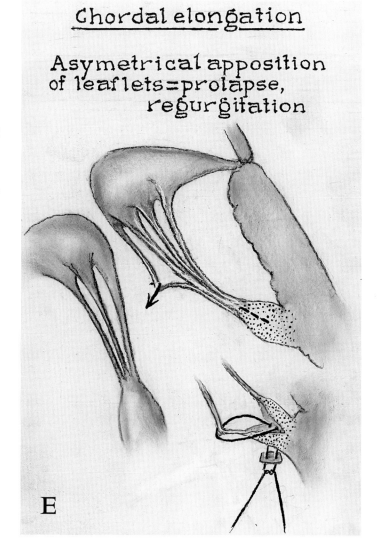

Chordal elongation

Asymetrical apposition of leaflets=prolapse, regurgitation

E

use neochordae in the form of 4-0 or 5-0 Gortex suture. The use of Gortex chordae and their long-term results have been elegantly described by Dr. Tirone David of Toronto. When using this technique, one begins by first placing a 4-0 or 5-0 Gortex suture with a pledget through the fibrous head of the given papillary muscle in a horizontal mattress fashion. The two ends of the sutures are subsequently passed through the free end of the given leaflet and tied to the proper length. This is determined by providing upward traction on the anterior leaflet at a height which is proportionate to a normal segment of the valve. This is most commonly done by comparison with the opposite leaflet, which is usually not plagued by long chordae. Such traction at the given height is maintained by engaging the free leaflet edge with either a nerve hook or other such instrument which will allow a firm knot to be placed without sliding the knot and excessively decreasing the length of the neochordae. The knot on the leaflet end may be reinforced with a pledget if the leaflet tissue is judged to be relatively thin. Such a technique can be applied for multiple chordae and positions, and we find this technique to be much faster and more reliable when chordal shortening is required.

F-G The single most common form of mitral valve repair involves ruptured chordae to one or both leaflets. The most common position for such rupture is in the central segment of the posterior leaflet. Again, this is commonly found in myxomatous disease and can be handled with a quadrangular excision. The area of the ruptured chordae is first isolated by passing a 2-0 silk suture around the intact chordae, which are on either side of the rupture chordae. These sutures are

placed on mild tension and thus define the line for the quadrangular resection. The ruptured chordae themselves are then grasped and a #15 blade is used to begin the incision into the posterior leaflet. This is carried through the leaflet to, but not into, the mitral annulus. The second incision is repeated on the opposite side of the ruptured chordae and that rectangle with its base at the mitral annulus is then extracted as shown in figure F. The base is subsequently sharply

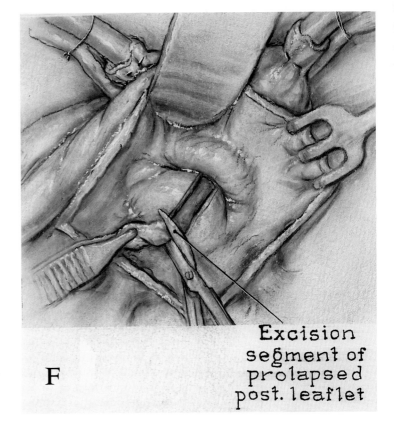

F

Excision
segment of
prolapsed
post. leaflet

F-G *continued*

divided from the annulus. The repair of the ensuing defect is begun with the plication of the annulus itself. This is done using a pledgeted 2-0 or 3-0 braided suture which is placed in the annulus near the end of the leaflet defect, and brought out beyond the opposite end of the defect. This suture is then tied, thus plicating the annulus in the area of the leaflet defect. The leaflet edges are then rejoined. My preference is to use a running 4-0 braided ticron suture, which is begun at the free end of the leaflet. The leaflet is then closed with a running suture which ends at the mitral annulus. The second limb of that suture is subsequently brought down in an opposite direction and tied at the annulus. Such a technique employs soft suture with the ends being tied at the annulus. Therefore, those ends are not exposed on the leaflet edges themselves. It is impossible to have those edges impinge or potentially damage the anterior leaflet during the normal excursion of the valve. Other techniques which have been described for leaflet closure involve using 5-0 prolene placed as individual sutures (usually 5–6 in number). While certainly effective in closing the leaflet, these stiffer ends of the prolene can theoretically injure the anterior leaflet during normal functioning of the valve. Finally, the quadrangular repair is reinforced by the use of an annuloplasty ring. Figure G shows a circumferential ring (a Duran ring) which has been placed with a running suture. The technique for placement of an annuloplasty ring is identical to that described in the earlier part of this chapter. Though the use of an annuloplasty ring for reinforcement is not mandatory in all forms of quadrangular repair, it is certainly recommended in that it removes tension from the suture line at the point of annular plication. Integrity of the repair is then tested using hand injections of saline into the LV cavity as described earlier in the chapter.

Such posterior rectangular excision can be used for up to 50% of the posterior leaflet. When larger segments of the posterior leaflets are resected, annular plication is not feasible and a technique of "sliding plasty" is required. This involves first removing the affected aspect of the posterior leaflet. It is followed by partial division of the remaining posterior leaflet from its annular attachment and subsequent reattachment of that segment of the leaflet with mattress sutures or a continuous stitch of 2-0 or 3-0 braided sutures. The posterior leaflet is advanced along the posterior annulus such that the two leaflet edges eventually reapproximate themselves, but the plication of the posterior annulus is achieved in a gradual fashion. The free edges are then reapproximated as describe above. Such an extensive repair definitely requires support with an annuloplasty ring.

Rupture chordae from the anterior leaflet may be repaired in one of two ways: (1) Artificial chordae using 4-0 or 5-0 Gortex sutures are constructed to replace the ruptured chordae. This technique was described previously in this chapter. (2) The ruptured chordae to the anterior leaflet may be replaced by

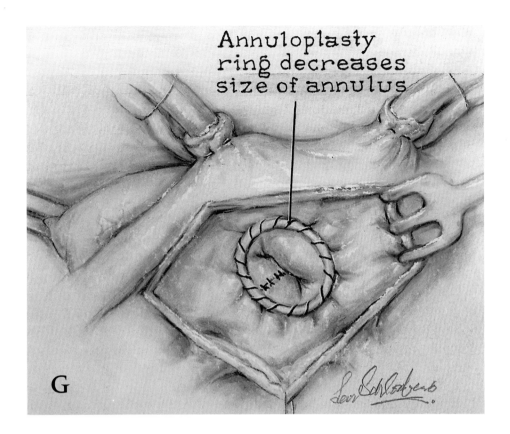

Annuloplasty
ring decreases
size of annulus

G

normal chordae from the posterior leaflet in the "flip over" technique. This involves performing a quadrangular excision of the posterior leaflet, which is opposite the corresponding ruptured chordae on the anterior leaflet. However, instead of removing the posterior leaflet and its chordae, they are retained, and the posterior leaflet is transposed onto the free edge of the anterior leaflet and secured in place using a 4-0 or 5-0 braided suture. The subsequent defect in the posterior leaflet is handled as described above, with posterior annular plication and leaflet reapproximation. Again, such a repair should be augmented by an annuloplasty ring.

Chapter 10

Removal of Myxoma

R. Scott Stuart, M.D.

Introduction

The majority of cardiac myxomas reside in the left atrium, although there are notable reports describing their existence in all cardiac chambers, including the ventricles. Nonetheless, the left atrial location predominates. Generally, a myxoma will arise on a pedicled stalk, which can be quite narrow (even 2–3 mm) or very broad and sessile. The majority of such attachments will be on the atrial septum. However, myxomas have been described as arising from various parts of the mitral valve apparatus. This chapter will describe the removal of myxomas from the atrium with the stalk arising from the atrial septum, since this approach potentially requires more repair than those arising from other locations.

A   Since most myxomas are found within the left atrium, the approach will be very similar that used in mitral valve procedures (see chapter drawings, Mitral Valve Approaches and Procedures). These drawings depict a right atrial approach with access to the left atrium gained through the atrial septum. Full details of this approach may be found within the mitral valve chapter. It is enough to say here that the approach through the right atrium is preceded by atrial double cannulation using Rumel tourniquets. The right atrium may be opened with either a vertical or a modified horizontal incision, with the goal being good exposure of the underlying fossa ovale. As is shown, the fossa is opened with an incision which extends from a superior to inferior direction, and it is most easily begun within the fossa in the region of the limbus. This incision is extended far enough to gain a good view of the left atrium, and exposure is augmented by the use of one or two vein retractors.

B   A myxoma with its pedicle arising from the inferior aspect of the divided atrial septum. As shown, the myxoma is not simply removed from its pedicle, rather the entire myxoma and stalk are removed with a collar of presumably normal septal tissue. The specimen is removed intact and sent to pathology.

C   The resulting defect may be as small as a few millimeters, but typically it is as large as one and, occasionally, two centimeters in diameter.

D   Subsequent repair of the atrial septostomy with its extended defect is most commonly completed with a pericardial patch which is easily available. The comfortably sized, usually circular patch is fashioned and, when sewn into the septal defect, is placed with the "shiny" surface facing the left atrium. The closure is most commonly performed with the patch first being secured in a triangular or quadrangular fashion with 4-0 prolene, and the intervening space between these sutures is closed with the running of the suture. The right atrium is closed in the standard fashion with a running 3-0 or 4-0 prolene suture.

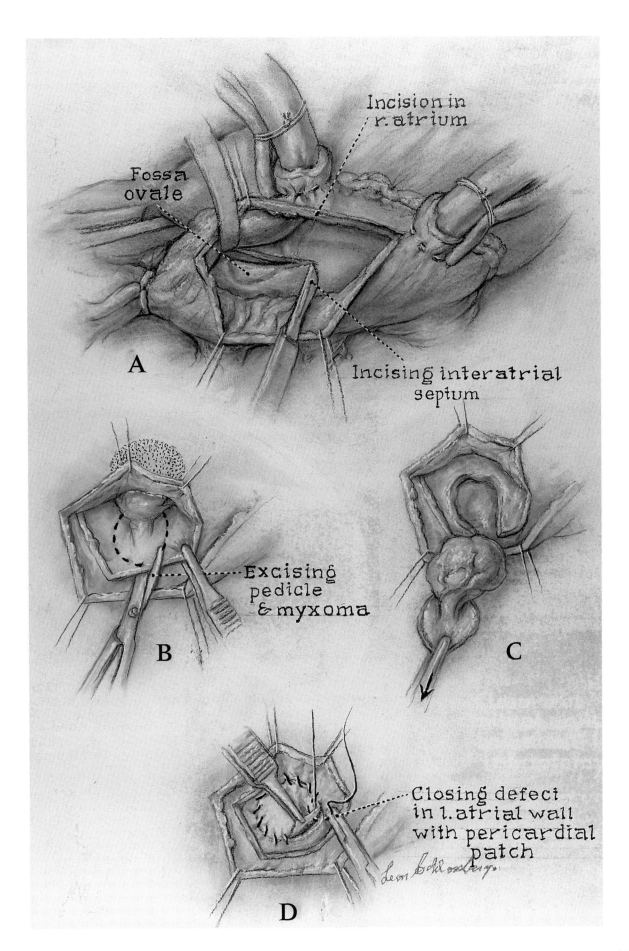

Incision in
r. atrium

Fossa
ovale

Incising interatrial
septum

A

Excising
pedicle
& myxoma

B

C

Closing defect
in l. atrial wall
with pericardial
patch

Leon Schlossberg

D

E-F The more common approach to the left atrium is directly into the left atrium via an incision just below Waterston's groove. The approach is identical to that used when addressing a mitral valve and is preceded by atrial double cannulation. Rumel tourniquets may or may not be employed depending on the preference of the surgeon. Full details of this incision are described in the mitral valve chapter.

G This figure represents the resection of a left atrial myxoma with removal of a collar of atrial septum along with the stalk and myxoma. Here the atrial septum has been everted to bring the septum and myxoma into the field. The mitral valve is hidden in the inferior aspect of the incision behind the myxoma.

H The resulting defect is closed primarily with a 3-0 or 4-0 prolene suture. If the defect is reasonably large, a pericardial patch may be employed as described above.

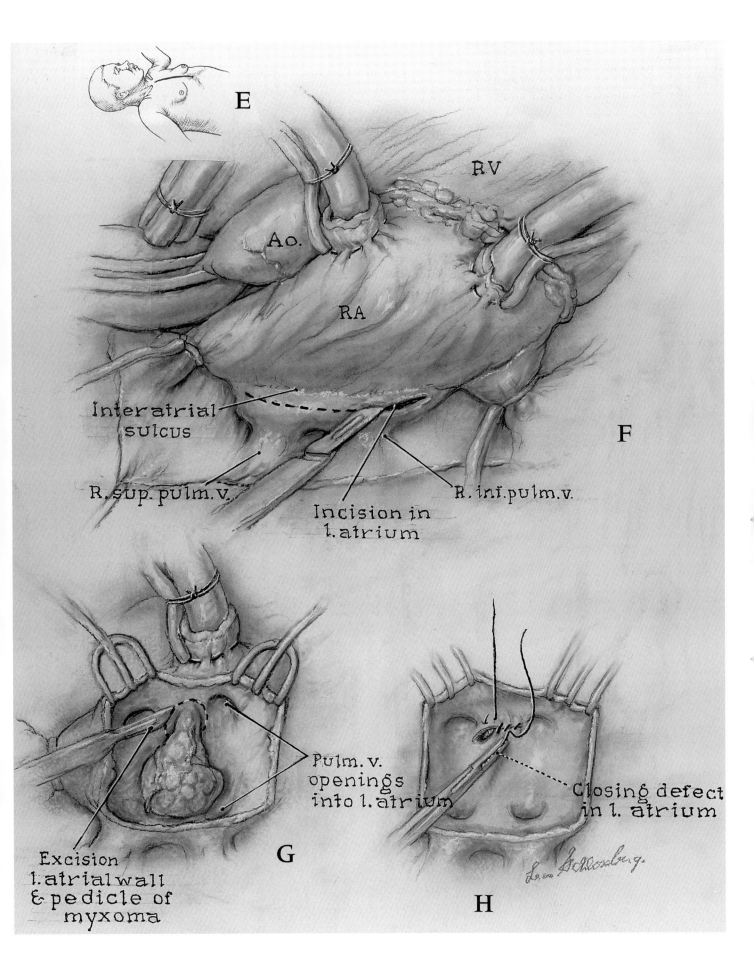

E

Ao.

RV

RA

Interatrial
sulcus

R. sup. pulm. v.

Incision in
l. atrium

R. inf. pulm. v.

F

Pulm. v.
openings
into l. atrium

G

Excision
l. atrial wall
& pedicle of
myxoma

Closing defect
in l. atrium

H

Chapter 11

The Standard Maze-III Procedure

James L. Cox, M.D.

Introduction

The original Maze procedure (Maze-I) was introduced clinically in September, 1987. Although this technique was extremely effective in controlling atrial fibrillation, it resulted in two unforseen problems:

1. Chronotropic inadequacy of the sinoatrial (SA) node.

   Many patients were unable to develop a sinus tachycardia rate commensurate with the level of their physical activity postoperatively because one of the incisions was positioned in the "sinus-tachycardia region" of the SA node, immediately anterior to the orifice of the superior vena cava (SVC).
2. Prolonged intra-atrial conduction delay.

   This resulted in the sinus node impulse arriving in the left atrium at the same time it arrived in the left ventricle. This, in turn, resulted in apparent absence of left atrial contraction postoperatively because it was contracting at the same time as the left ventricle.

Because of these problems in the first 32 patients, the Maze-I procedure was modified to the Maze-II procedure in the next 15 patients. This technique was equally effective in controlling atrial fibrillation but proved to be extremely difficult to perform because of the frequent necessity for transection of the SVC. As a result, the Maze-II was further modified to the Maze-III procedure, which is depicted in the following figures. This technique has been in continuous use since April, 1992 and, therefore, has been used in the vast majority of patients in our series. Both problems mentioned above were abolished by this last modification in technique.

A After aortic and bicaval cannulation for cardiopulmonary bypass, the left ventricle is vented through the right pulmonary vein. The aorta is cross-clamped and the heart is cardioplegically arrested. The right atrial appendage is excised, leaving a left atrial muscle "bridge" of at least 2 cm between the base of the excised appendage and the superior vena cava (SVC). Note the approximate position of the sinoatrial (S-A) node.

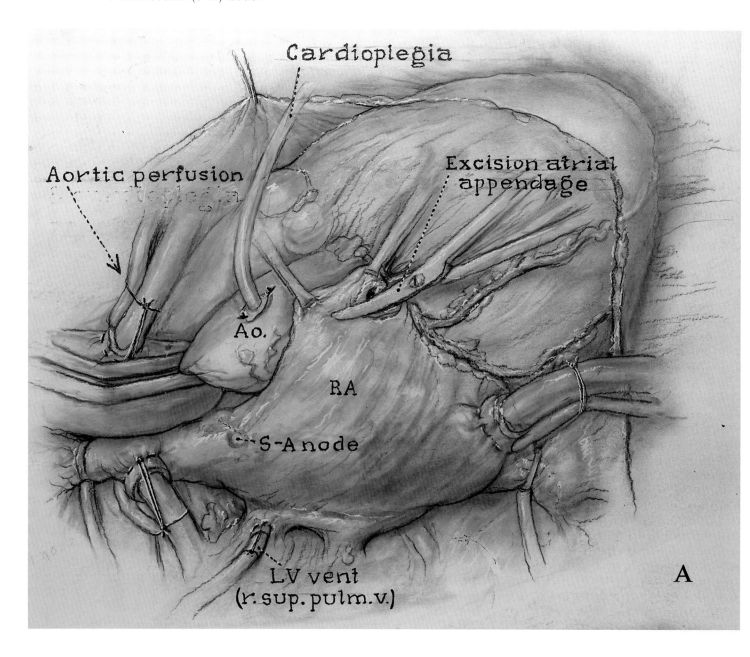

B   Following excision of the right atrial appendage, a short lateral atriotomy is extended downward from the appendage for 2-3 cm and a cardiotomy suction is inserted into the cavity of the right atrium. A long posterior atriotomy is then placed from the SVC to the IVC staying well posterior to the site of the S-A node.

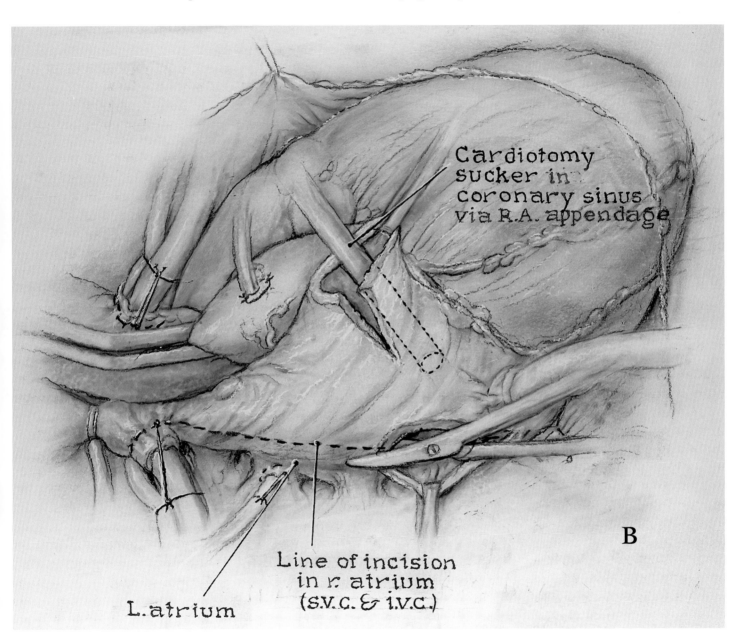

Cardiotomy sucker in coronary sinus via R.A. appendage

B

L. atrium

Line of incision in r. atrium (s.v.c. & i.v.c.)

C   A "T" incision is placed from the posterior atriotomy to the top of the A-V groove on the right atrial free-wall. This incision should be at least 1 cm above the IVC cannula and at least 3 cm below the short lateral atriotomy that extends from the base of the right atrial appendage.

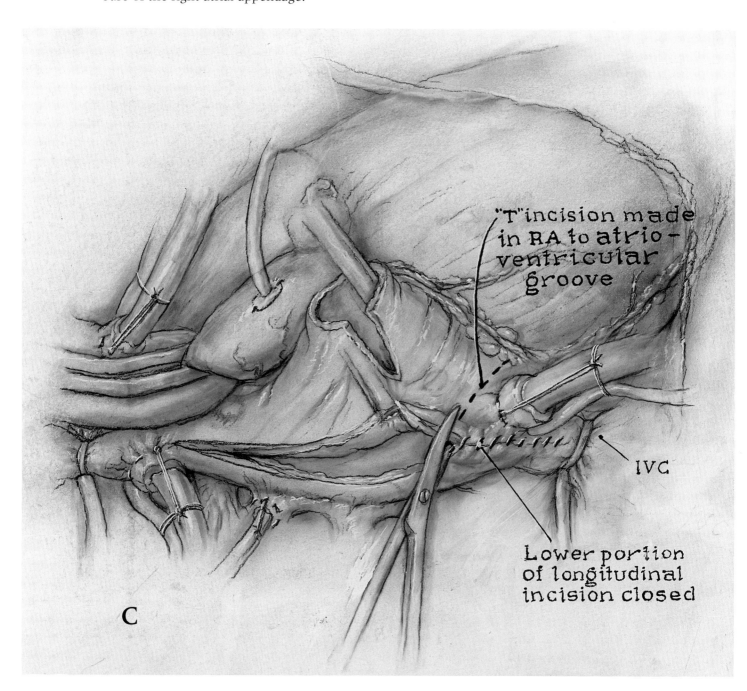

"T" incision made in RA to atrio-ventricular groove

IVC

Lower portion of longitudinal incision closed

C

D The free-wall of the right atrium is retracted superiorly to expose the inside of the right atrium. The T incision is then extended to the level of the tricuspid annulus well anterior to the os of the coronary sinus. This should be a transmural incision through the muscle of the right atrial wall underlying the fat pad of the A-V groove but not through the A-V groove itself because the latter harbors the right coronary artery.

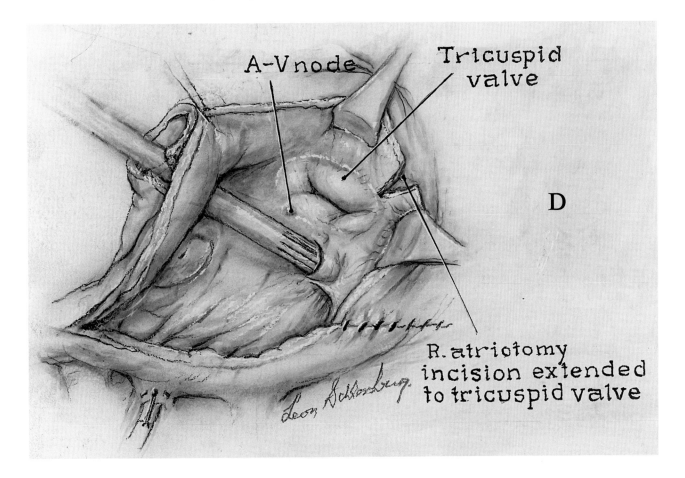

A-V node

Tricuspid valve

D

R. atriotomy incision extended to tricuspid valve

E   To ensure that all conduction across the T incision is interrupted, all visible reddish myocardial fibers must be dissected away from the A-V groove fat pad. This is best accomplished with a small nerve hook.

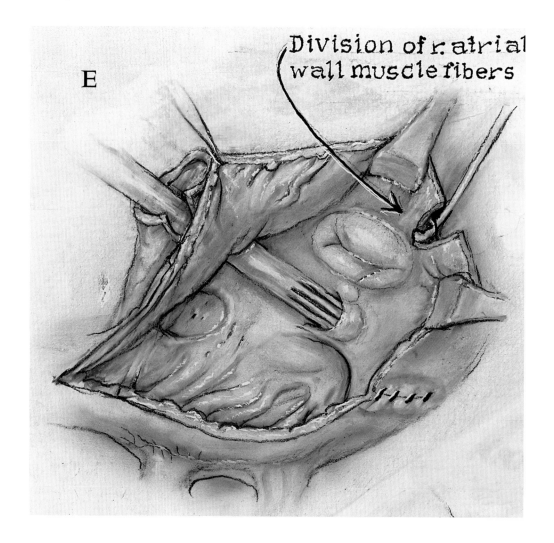

F   A two-millimeter cryolesion is placed at the end of the T incision at the level of the tricuspid valve annulus to be certain that no conduction can occur across the T incision because of undetected myocardial fibers that may reside near the annulus.

G   The lower portion of the T incision beneath the fat pad of the A-V groove is closed with 4-0 polypropylene suture. The counter incision (dashed line) is placed from the anterior-medial base of the excised right atrial appendage down to the level of the tricuspid valve annulus. This incision is well anterior to the A-V node when it intersects the annulus.

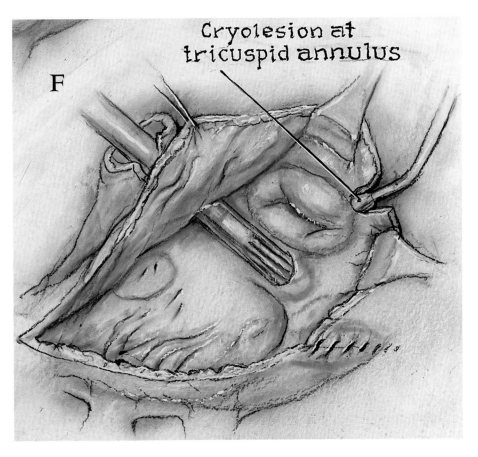

Cryolesion at tricuspid annulus

F

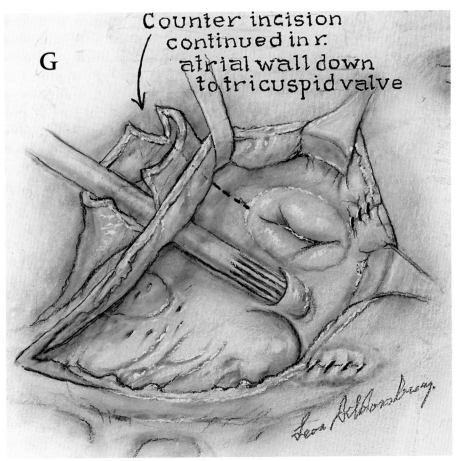

Counter incision continued in r. atrial wall down to tricuspid valve

G

H A two-millimeter cryolesion is placed at the lower end of the counter incision to preclude any conduction across this region near the tricuspid valve annulus.

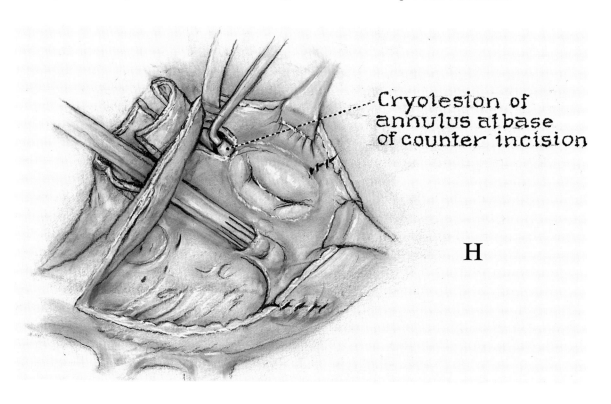

I The counter incision is closed with 4-0 polypropylene suture.

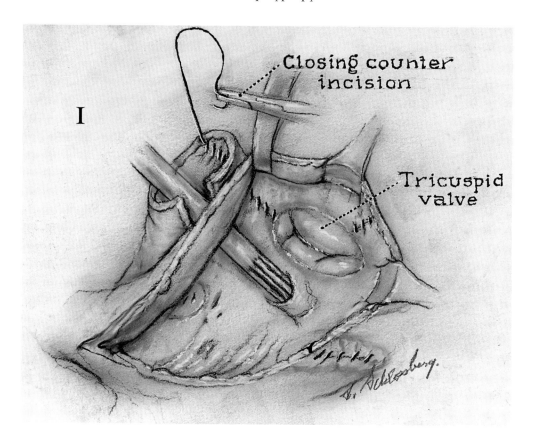

J   A standard left atriotomy is placed in the inter-atrial groove. The atrial septum is then divided (dashed line) across the anterior limbus of the fossa ovalis and across the fossa ovalis itself. Note that this atrial septotomy is placed well posterior to the orifice of the SVC.

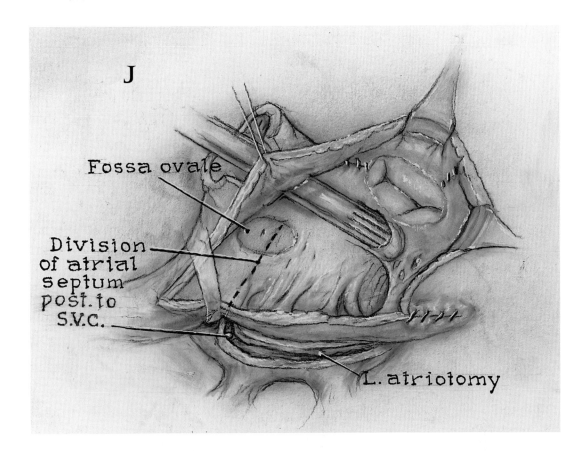

K The standard left atriotomy is extended both superiorly and inferiorly toward the orifices of the left superior and left inferior pulmonary veins and then along the ridge (dashed line) that separates the pulmonary vein orifices from the orifice of the left atrial appendage. The two ends of this pulmonary-vein-encircling incision should **not** be made to meet because the pulmonary veins may retract and make the subsequent alignment and closure difficult.

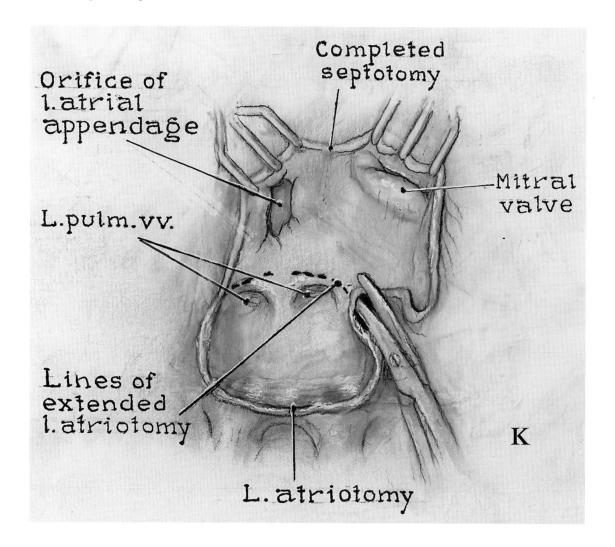

L The entire left atrial appendage is inverted into the inside of the left atrial cavity and excised along its base. This is done carefully with a small scalpel, taking care not to injure the circumflex coronary artery. Note the bridge of atrium remaining between the two ends of the pulmonary-vein-encircling incision.

M The bridge of tissue between the two ends of the pulmonary-vein-encircling incision and at the base of the excised left atrial appendage is cryoablated to complete the electrical isolation of all four pulmonary vein orifices.

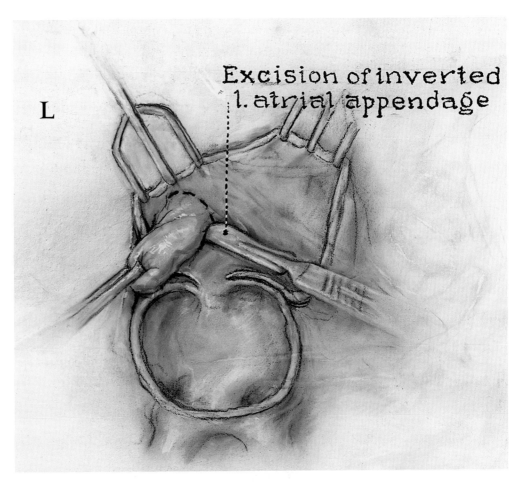

Excision of inverted
l. atrial appendage

L

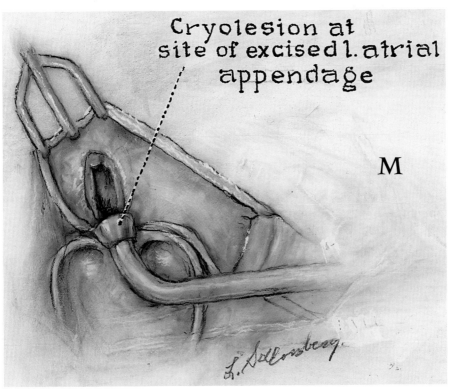

Cryolesion at
site of excised l. atrial
appendage

M

N The base of the excised left atrial appendage is closed with a 4-0 polypropylene suture. A posterior-vertical incision is placed between the pulmonary-vein-encircling incision and the middle of the posterior mitral valve annulus. This is a transmural incision through the myocardium of the left atrium but **not** through the A-V groove fat pad, which harbors the circumflex coronary artery and the coronary sinus.

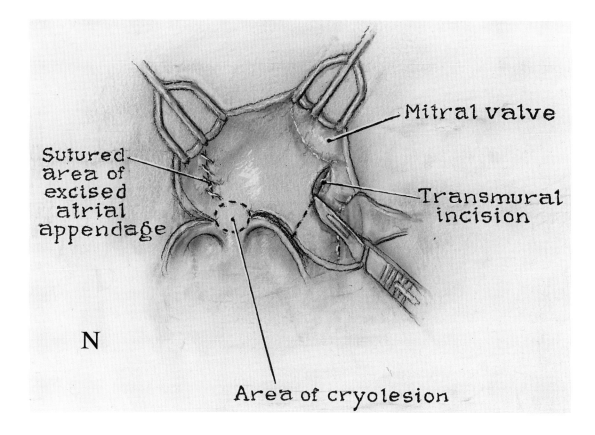

O A nerve hook is used to divide any remaining small muscle fibers overlying the A-V groove fat pad, and the coronary sinus is then cryoablated circumferentially. We use a right-angled cryoprobe and place it behind the coronary sinus (i.e., on its epicardial surface) so that we can be certain that the cryolesion in the coronary sinus is indeed circumferential.

P A two-millimeter cryolesion is placed at the mitral end of the posterior-vertical left atriotomy to block any possible conduction at the level of the annulus.

Q The posterior-vertical left atriotomy is closed with a 4-0 polypropylene suture. Most recurrences arise from electrical conduction that is reestablished across this incision line (or via the coronary sinus). Therefore, we usually place metal vascular clips in the edges of this incision as we close it to provide a radiographic marker to guide placement of a radiofrequency catheter lesion in the event of a recurrence. The inferior and superior portions of the pulmonary-vein-encircling incision are then closed with 4-0 polypropylene suture.

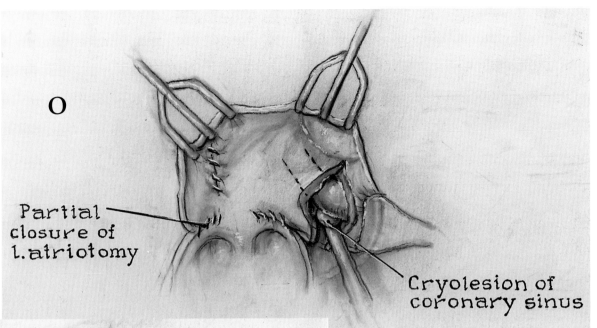

O

Partial
closure of
l. atriotomy

Cryolesion of
coronary sinus

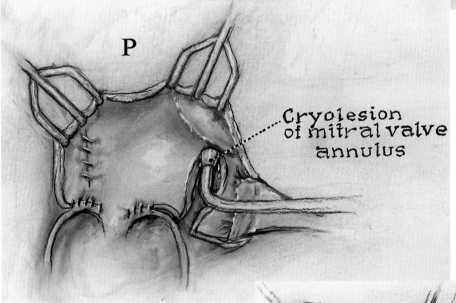

P

Cryolesion
of mitral valve
annulus

Closure of
mitral annulus
incision & l.
atriotomy

L. Schlossberg

Q

R The atrial septotomy closure begins at the lower end of the incision through the fossa ovalis.

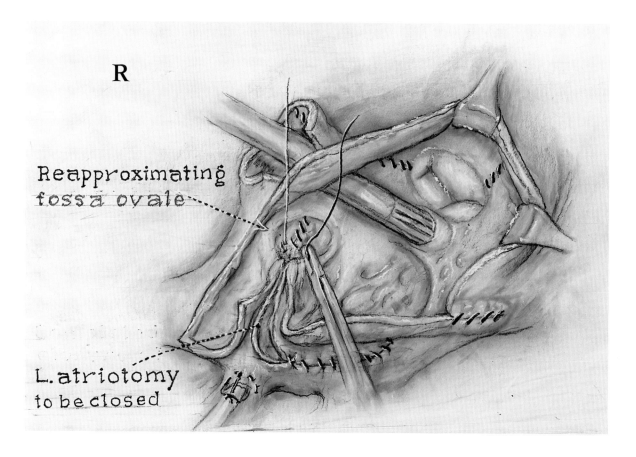

S Just prior to complete closure of the two ends of the left atriotomy (i.e., the pulmonary-vein-encircling incision), the atrial septotomy is closed. The fossa ovalis is closed in one layer that is contiguous with the posterior (left atrial) side of the thick anterior limbus.

T Once the left atrium is closed, the anterior (right atrial) side of the thick anterior limbus is closed with a separate 4-0 polypropylene suture.

U Appearance of the heart following completion of the Maze procedure and removal of all cardiopulmonary bypass cannulae.

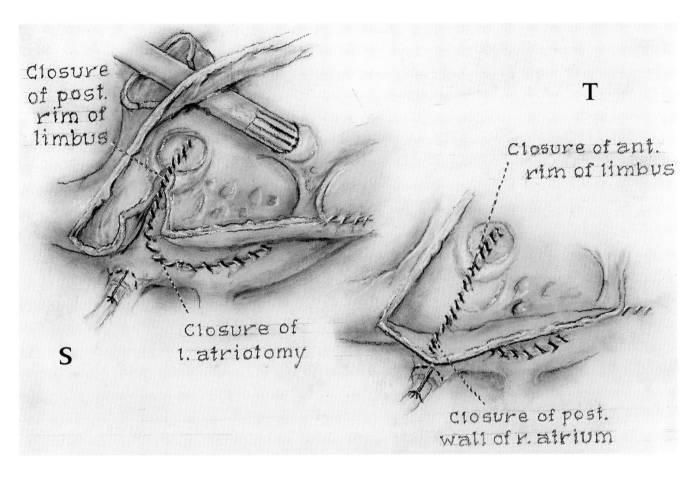

Closure of post. rim of limbus

T

Closure of ant. rim of limbus

Closure of l. atriotomy

S

Closure of post. wall of r. atrium

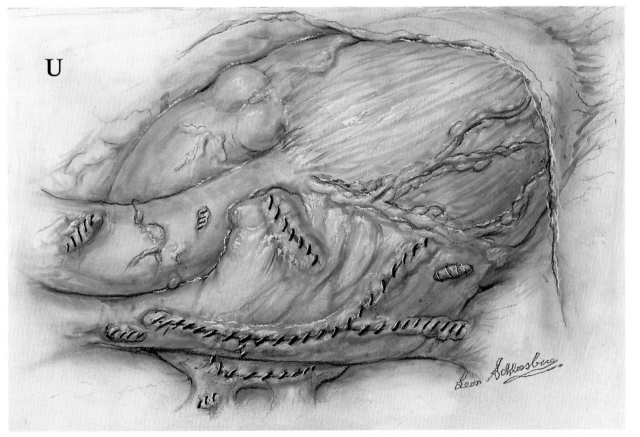

U

Chapter 12

Hypertrophic Obstructive Cardiomyopathy

William A. Baumgartner, M.D.

Introduction

Hypertrophic obstructive cardiomyopathy (HOCM) is a familial disease associated with autosomal-dominant inheritance and characterized grossly by myocardial hypertrophy and microscopically by a disorganization of the cardiomyocytes. Approximately 25% of patients have a dynamic obstructive component caused by a combination of factors, including systolic anterior motion (SAM), a narrowed outflow tract, and rapid ventricular ejection. Symptoms and signs associated with hypertrophic cardiomyopathy are manifested by diastolic dysfunction, dysrhythmias (atrial and ventricular), myocardial ischemia, and congestive heart failure. The primary long-term cause of death is dysrhythmias.

Treatment consists of prevention of congestive heart failure and control of dysrhythmias. There is an outflow tract gradient in a quarter of patients for whom medical interventions such as beta blockers, disopyramide, and calcium antagonists can improve symptoms.

When drug therapy fails, newer nonsurgical approaches have included pacing and alcohol ablation. A number of studies have demonstrated that duel-chamber pacing with a short AV delay promotes constant activation of the right ventricle from its apex and thereby relieves the outflow tract gradient. Alcohol ablation is a catheter-based technique in which alcohol is injected into the first septal perforator or branch of the left anterior descending coronary artery. This technique has been used in only a limited number of patients, but the preliminary data suggest that there is significant gradient reduction.

Operative intervention is considered when these nonsurgical methods have failed and the patient continues to have an outflow gradient of > 50 mmHg with associated symptoms. The primary aim of surgical intervention is to eliminate SAM by increasing the left ventricular outflow tract dimension.

The anatomic hallmark of HOCM is asymmetrical left ventricular hypertrophy with marked enlargement (> 2 cm) of the intraventricular septum which appears predominantly just inferior to the right coronary leaflet of the aortic valve. The operation of choice is a ventricular septal myotomy and myectomy (M&M) originally described and performed by Dr. Andrew G. Morrow. This classic operation is infrequently performed today as the majority of patients with HOCM can be treated medically or with other novel therapeutic interventions. Operative mortality associated with this operation is approximately 1 to 2%. Complications include atrial-ventricular block, ventricular septal defect, and acute aortic regurgitation. Further work at the National Institutes of Health demonstrated that when the ventricular septum is less than 2 cm in thickness, the primary operation should be mitral valve replacement. It was felt that a septal thickness less than 2 cm would increase the chances of producing a ventricular septal defect using the standard myotomy-myectomy approach.

The following figures depict the classic myotomy-myectomy operation as originally described by Dr. Morrow. Dr. Morrow mentored Dr. Edward Stinson from Stanford, who then instructed me on the procedure.

Anesthesia. For patients with hypertrophic obstructive cardiomyopathy, the use of any type of pressor agent is contraindicated. These agents cause an increased in contractility, thereby increasing the outflow tract gradient. In addition, d-tubocurarine should also be avoided in these patients since its action of ganglionic blockade can result in hypotension. If hypotension does occur, the drug of choice is phenylephrine, with volume loading.

A   Incision and Exposure

A standard median sternotomy is made. The setup is similar to an aortic valve operation. A dual-stage venous cannula and standard central aortic cannulation are used. A left atrial vent is placed through the right superior pulmonary vein. Several options are available for myocardial protection. I still employ a single antegrade bolus of crystalloid cardioplegia followed by a topical hypothermia using pericardial lavage with 4° C saline. Systemic temperature is maintained at approximately 30° C.

Exposure of the aortic valve and interventricular septum is through an oblique aortotomy extended into the area of the non-coronary sinus. The pericardial stay sutures are generally not placed on the left-hand side so that the left ventricle is posterior, giving maximum exposure to the ventricular septum. For myocardial preservation purposes, it also allows cold saline to completely cover the left ventricle and most of the right ventricle.

The ventricular septum is exposed by a combination of maneuvers. First, an assistant, using a sponge stick, depresses the anterior wall of the right ventricle, thereby pushing the ventricular septum into view. This is not always necessary since gentle retraction of the right coronary leaflet is often adequate to expose the ventricular septum.

The ventricular septum is checked for any scarring caused by the trauma associated with the anterior segment of the mitral valve. In addition, the mitral valve is examined for any abnormalities. A transesophageal echo is a very useful adjunct. In addition to confirming the location of the asymmetric thickness of the septum, it defines any abnormalities of the mitral valve itself. Following the repair, it provides information regarding the adequacy of repair. Specifically, it identifies the "trench" that is made with the myotomy and myectomy. In addition, it will identify whether there is any SAM remaining and the degree of mitral regurgitation, if any.

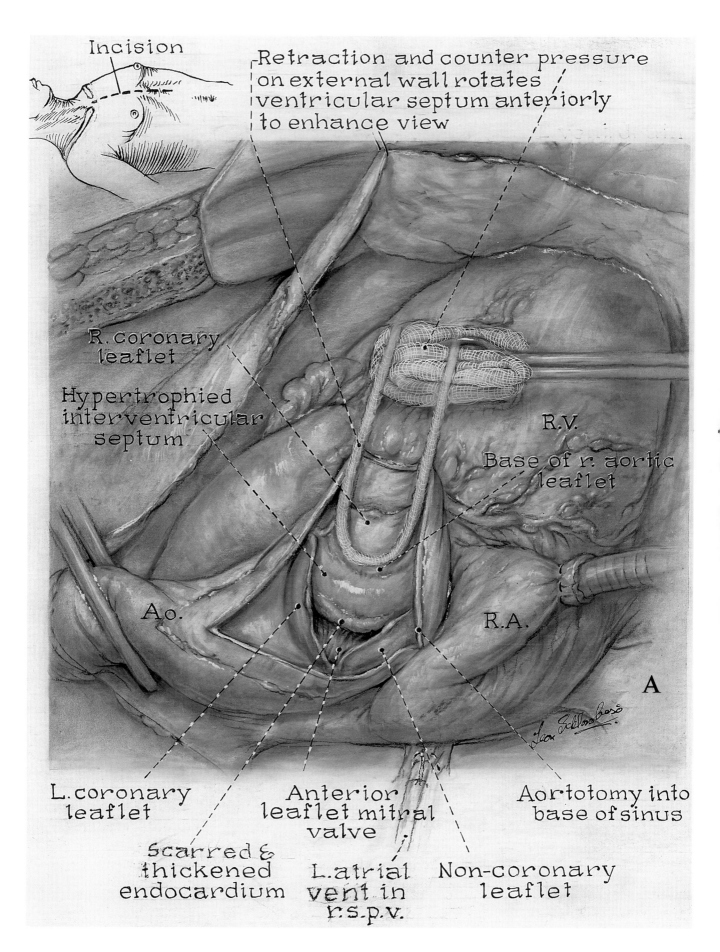

Incision

Retraction and counter pressure on external wall rotates ventricular septum anteriorly to enhance view

R. coronary leaflet

Hypertrophied interventricular septum

R.V.

Base of r. aortic leaflet

Ao.

R.A.

A

L. coronary leaflet

Anterior leaflet mitral valve

Aortotomy into base of sinus

Scarred & thickened endocardium

L. atrial vent in r.s.p.v.

Non-coronary leaflet

A ribbon retractor is bent in a gentle S curve to provide protection to the mitral valve and its posterior apparatus while the myotomy is being performed. It is also helpful to place a moist sponge in the outflow track area to assist with displacing the mitral valve and papillary muscles inferior to the retractor. Generally, retractors in the size range of 16–20 mm provide adequate coverage without injuring the aortic valve leaflets.

B-C Myectomy Incisions

The first vertical incision is placed just to the right of center of the right coronary leaflet. By keeping the incision in this location, the membranous portion of the septum is as well as the atrioventricular node are to the right of this area. Using Dr. Morrow's instruments that are angled to prevent obscuring the view of the septum during the myotomy, the blade is directed parallel to the ribbon retractor. This first vertical incision is extended to the apex for the entire length of the 10 blade as well as up to ~ 1 cm of the handle. Once inserted, it is then directed posteriorly in a cutting fashion until it abuts the ribbon retractor. Before any myotomy incisions are made, the cordal apparatus is checked to be sure it is all posterior to the ribbon retractor.

D Longitudinal View of Myotomy

This longitudinal view of the heart demonstrates the angle of the knife blade being inserted in a vertical manner. It also demonstrates the curve of the ribbon retractor so that the 10 blade will abut it during the actual cutting motion. With the left atrial vent in place, the exposure is generally adequate, allowing reasonably good visualization of the ventricular septum.

E Completion of the Myotomy Incisions

A second vertical incision is made in the same manner approximately 1 cm to the left of the first incision. The third incision is made transversely, connecting the two vertical incisions. It is begun approximately 2 mm below the annulus of the right coronary leaflet. Similar to the vertical incisions, this incision needs to be parallel to the septum and the ribbon retractor. The depth of this incision should be similar to that made with the vertical myotomies so as to remove the entire portion of ventricular septum.

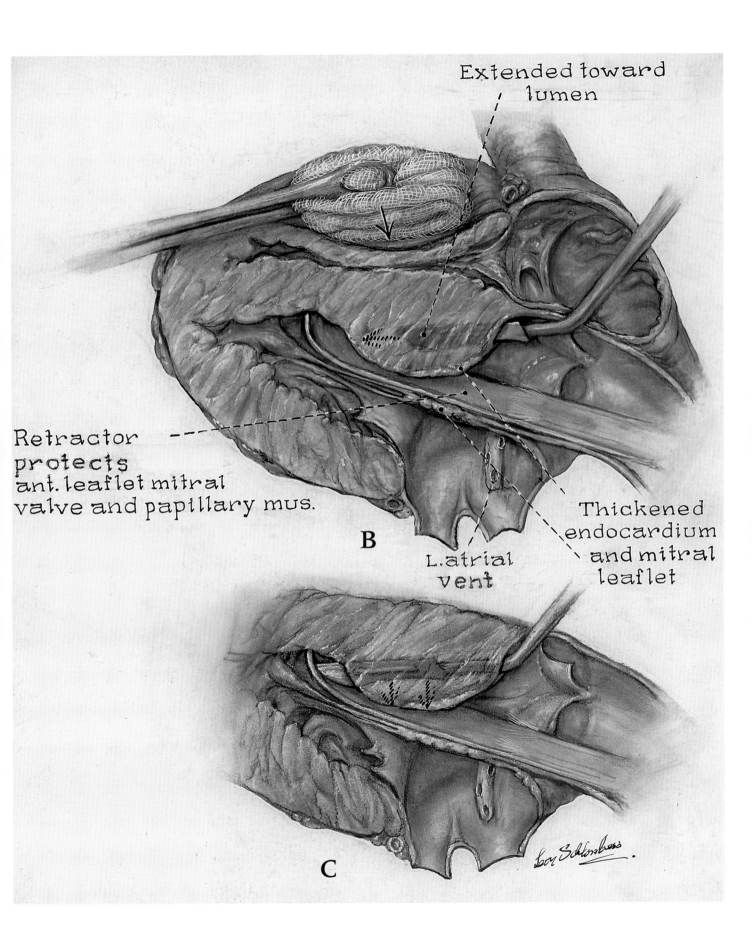

Extended toward lumen

Retractor protects ant. leaflet mitral valve and papillary mus.

B

L. atrial vent

Thickened endocardium and mitral leaflet

C

Leon Schlossberg.

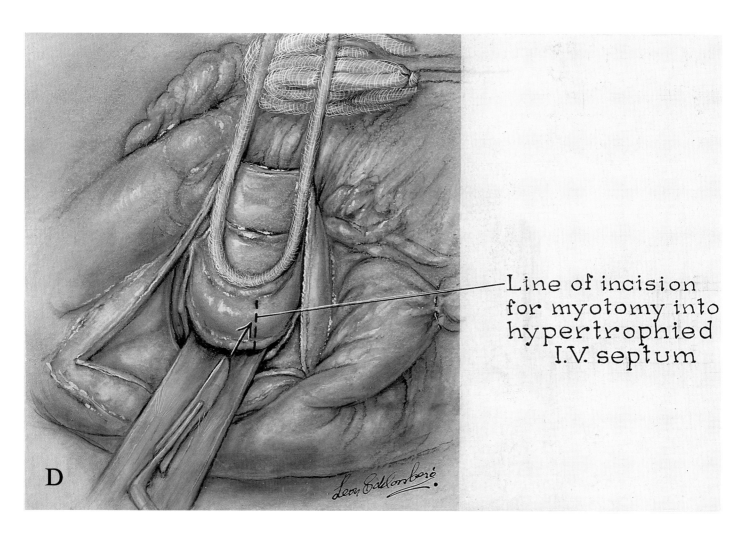

Line of incision
for myotomy into
hypertrophied
I.V. septum

D

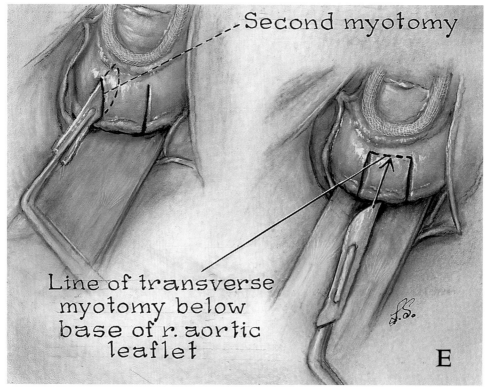

Second myotomy

Line of transverse
myotomy below
base of r. aortic
leaflet

E

F   Segment of Muscle Removed

The myotomy and myectomy generally results in a crescent-shaped portion of muscle, containing scar on the endocardial surface. Fine-tipped scissors are often used to complete the myectomy. If the myotomy incisions made with the 10 blade have been adequate, this portion of muscle can be removed without fragmentation.

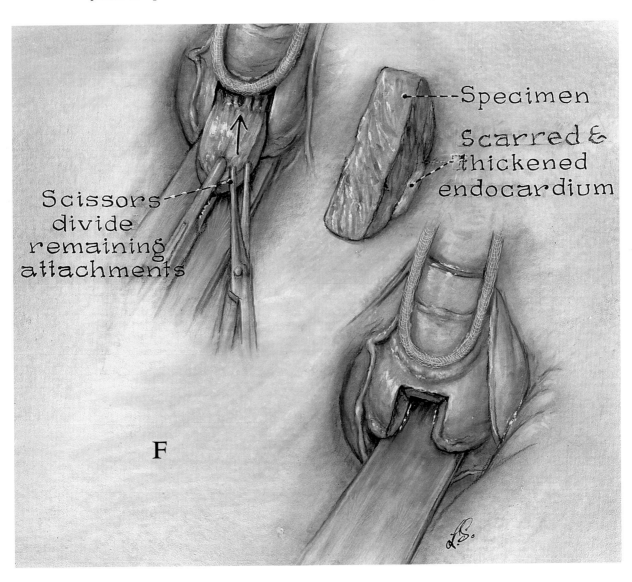

G Tailoring of the M&M

The opening of the trough is often increased by dividing a portion of the muscle and thickened endocardium, particularly on the right side.

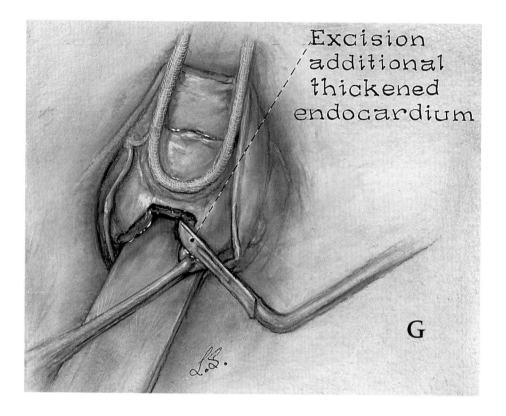

Excision additional thickened endocardium

G

H Completed Operation

The trough has been created under the right coronary leaflet and extended downward approximately to the mid-level of the ventricular septum. By keeping the first vertical incision just to the right, at the midportion of the right coronary leaflet, the AV node and membranous portion of the septum can be avoided.

Weaning the patient from cardiopulmonary bypass is generally not a challenge if adequate myocardial preservation has been maintained. Adequate volume loading as assessed by transesophageal echo generally is sufficient for separation from cardiopulmonary bypass. If vasodilatation has occurred, an infusion of phenylephrine is used.

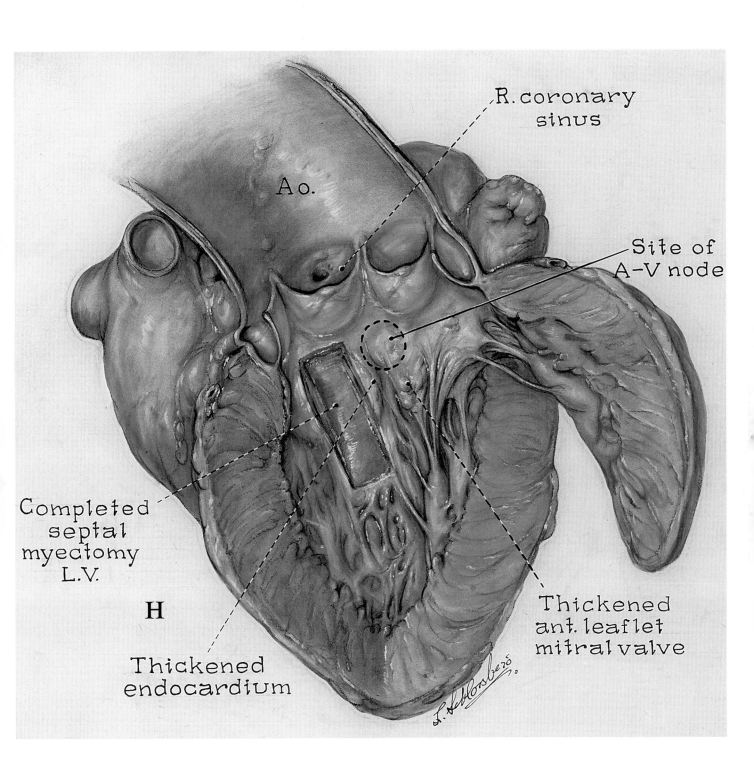

R. coronary sinus

Ao.

Site of A-V node

Completed septal myectomy L.V.

H

Thickened endocardium

Thickened ant. leaflet mitral valve

Chapter 13

Aortic Valve Replacement

R. Scott Stuart, M.D.

Introduction

Aortic valve replacement for aortic stenosis and/or aortic insufficiency is a fairly common and reasonably standard operation. As with the mitral valve, the choices for replacement valves are basically tissue or mechanical. Differences in implantation technique between these two valves are minor and will be described below. The physiology in aortic stenosis may be mimicked by valvular stenosis, supravalvular stenosis, or subvalvular stenosis, including problems with idiopathic hypertrophic subaortic stenosis (IHSS) and systolic anterior motion of the mitral valve. Only valve replacement related to valvular stenosis will be addressed in this chapter.

A   The patient is placed on cardiopulmonary bypass in the standard manner. Arterial cannulation is usually by way of the distal ascending aorta or proximal aortic arch, and venous cannulation is by way of the right atrium using a two-stage cannula. This figure illustrates the use of the pulmonary artery vent, which is commonly employed. My personal preference, whenever the left side of the heart is open, is to use a vent placed in the right superior pulmonary vein. This should reduce the entrapment of air in the pulmonary venous system from the open left side of the heart (which is possible with the use of a pulmonary artery vent). The other maneuver we frequently employ is the use of carbon dioxide, which is piped into the field with one-quarter inch tubing at a rate of 7 liters per minute. This should reduce the amount of air which will enter the left side of the heart, since the heavier CO_2 will displace air.

Once bypass is satisfactorily established and the vent is placed, the aortic cross-clamp may be applied. In cases of aortic insufficiency, where there are still significant amounts of volume being ejected by the left ventricle, it is best to wait until the heart fibrillates with the cooling of cardiopulmonary bypass. At that moment of fibrillation the cross-clamp is applied and the aorta opened. This avoids the expulsion of blood into the field from a beating heart which has been loaded with its regurgitant refraction.

The aortotomy is made with the initial incision being placed in the mid to left anterolateral aspect of the ascending aorta approximately one third of the distance along the ascending aorta as measured from the base of the aorta. Care must be taken not to make the aortotomy too close to the right coronary artery, thus compromising the ostium on subsequent closure of the aortotomy. The incision itself can be made in a vertical fashion as is somewhat depicted in this figure. Most commonly we employ a curvilinear incision (barber-pole like) which begins in the mid to left lateral ascending aorta and is carried downward in a curving fashion with the end of the aortotomy being directed toward the noncoronary sinus, and ending near the non- and left coronary commisure. Such an incision allows the aorta to unfold, which generally gives better exposure to the underlying valve. It also allows for the potential extension of the aortotomy into the commisural region, across 6the aortic anulus, and even into the left atrium should a Manugien type aortic root enlargement be necessary.

B-C   Exposure of the valve is augmented by placing stay sutures in the aortic wall as is depicted in Figure B. The valve is visually and manually inspected to determine the amount of calcification, and the leaflets are then sharply removed. The original leaflet resection is somewhat conservative to avoid breaching aortic-ventricular continuity. After the bulk of the stenotic valve is removed, one may return and do further sharp and even blunt debridement of the anulus either with scissors or small rongeurs. It is important that all anular calcium be removed to avoid the possibility of future periprosthetic leaks, which may be engendered by the gradual erosion of calcium trapped within the anular suture line. Frequently, only enough calcium is removed to allow penetration of a valve suture needle. While this is adequate for the immediate operation, it may do a

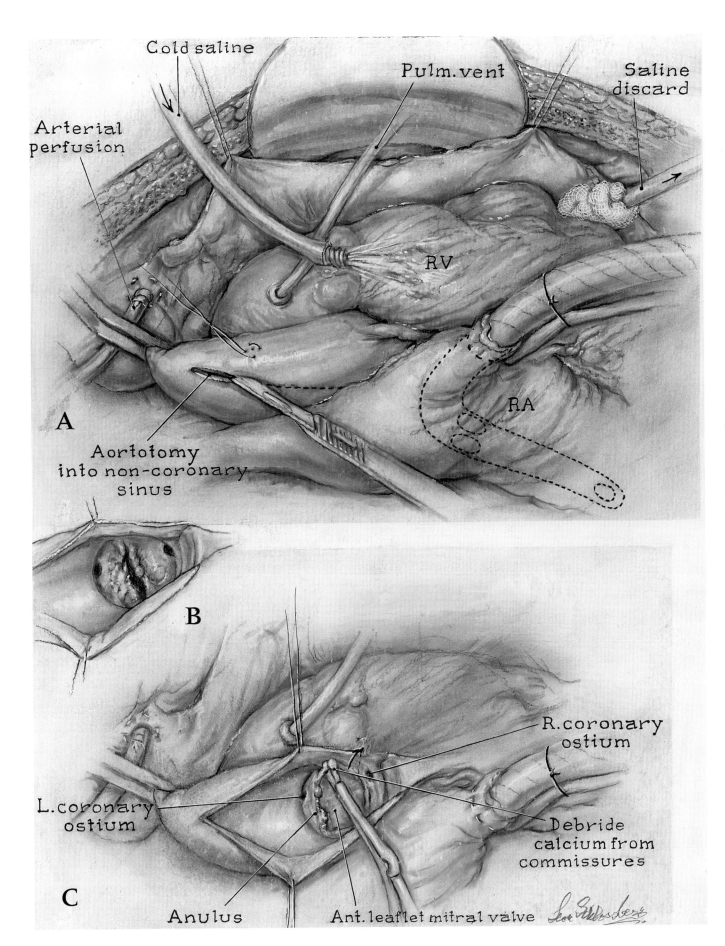

A

Cold saline

Arterial perfusion

Pulm. vent

Saline discard

RV

RA

Aortotomy into non-coronary sinus

B

C

L. coronary ostium

Anulus

Ant. leaflet mitral valve

R. coronary ostium

Debride calcium from commissures

disservice to the patient in terms of future periprosthetic leaks, which we have seen occur in 3 to 20 years following valve replacement. After the anulus is completely debrided, the aortic sinuses, anulus, and left ventricle are irrigated with saline solution to loosen and remove stray debris. Great care must be taken to adequately aspirate the anulus and ventricle to ensure that no potential calcium emboli will escape into the circulation following the completion of the operation. We prefer to use a metal yankauer with the screw-on tip removed for suction. This effectively creates a vacuum-like attachment which is excellent for retrieving small-to-moderate-sized pieces of calcium.

D After the anulus has been evaluated, the appropriate valve sutures are placed through the anulus itself.

E Sutures (usually a 2-0 braided suture with or without pledgets) are placed through the anulus. I have never been dogmatic in the method of suture placement. I am not married to an everting or "boiler plate" method of placement. I do recommend the use of horizontal mattress sutures but will either evert or come from below the anulus depending on the anatomy itself and the type of artificial valve employed. Commonly, everting techniques are preferred for mechanical valves because anular tissue is effectively removed from any potential leaflet impingement. Tissue valves do not suffer from such a danger and do equally well with an everting or a boiler plate technique. Likewise, pledgets may or may not be employed depending on the quality of the anulus and the aorta. My philosophy is, if the anulus is in good condition, the less artificial material within the root the better. Again, valve sutures are placed usually with a horizontal mattress technique with the mattress sutures themselves being separated only by a micromillimeter. The space within the suture placement is roughly five millimeters. The one critical point for great care is at the commisure between the right and coronary cusps. Here lies the membranous septum and its underlying conduction system. Deep bites in this area will run the risk of compromising the AV node and upper bundle and thus induce subsequent postoperative heart block. After the sutures are placed they may be secured by suture guides or (my preference) may be fanned out in a sunburst pattern across the operative field with the ends of the sutures being secured by straight clamps.

F After all sutures are placed through the anulus, the artificial valve is brought into the operative field. Depicted here is a tissue valve. As shown, the three struts of the tissue valve are often aligned with prior commisural positions of the native aortic valve. Mechanical valves obviously contain no such natural division, and frequently we will use a marking pen on the sewing ring to divide the circular apparatus into thirds or quadrants. Some mechanical valves actually come with prepackaged markers already applied to the sewing ring.

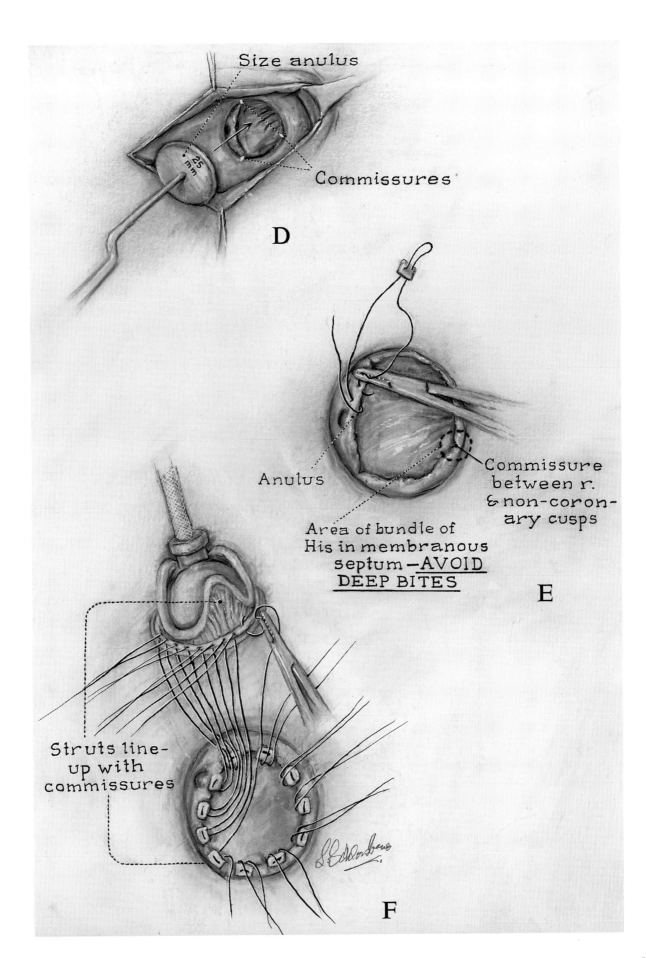

Size anulus

25 m m

Commissures

D

Anulus

Commissure between r. & non-coron-ary cusps

Area of bundle of His in membranous septum —AVOID DEEP BITES

E

Struts line-up with commissures

F

G After all sutures have been passed through the sewing ring of the artificial valve, the valve is lowered into place and excellent seating ensured as the sutures are tied with alternative throws crating a square knot. A total of six throws is usually sufficient for sutures made of braided material. After the valve is seated and all sutures have been tied, the ends of the sutures are cut, leaving tails of approximately 2 millimeters in length; this is long enough that the knots will not have a tendency to untie themselves but also short enough so that they will not interfere with mechanical valve leaflet function or engender a "whipping action" against the tissue valve's leaflet. After the valve sutures have been divided, final inspection is made of the valve itself to ensure that excellent seating has been obtained and that leaflet motion (especially for a mechanical valve) is free and unhindered. Additionally, final inspection is made of the aortic sinuses and coronary ostia to ensure that no stray pieces of calcium have found their way into those critical areas. A last look is made in the region where the aortic cross-clamp is placed. Often a small shelf is artificially created by the cross-clamp and can act as a repository for stray calcium pieces.

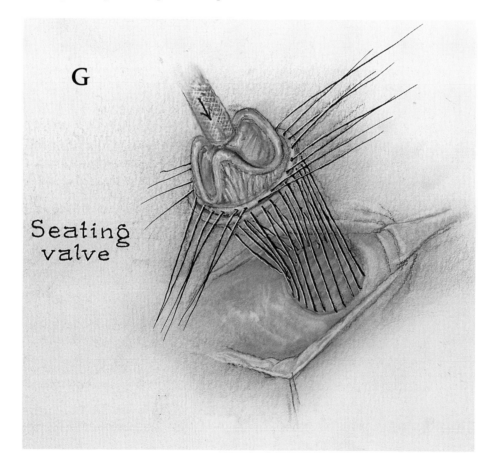

G

Seating
valve

H The aortotomy is closed with a running prolene suture. We prefer to use a running 3-0 or 4-0 prolene on an SH needle. My personal preference is to employ a running horizontal mattress suture as a first layer of closure. This allows for a very nice eversion of the aortic edges and provides a horizontal line of tension which is excellent in maintaining suture-line integrity in the postoperative period. This technique is followed by an over-and-over suture which passes through the everted edges of the aorta and stays above the line of the horizontal mattress suture. During the closure of the aortotomy, the vent is usually turned off and the ventricle passively filled with blood. If there still is an open space above the aortotomy at the point of final closure, some volume is taken from the pump and the lungs are inflated to further expel any air which may be entrapped within the pulmonary venous system. At this point the patient is placed in deep Trendelenburg position, and the final aspect of the aortic suture line is closed. Prior to removal of the cross-clamp, a dearing site is chosen on the ascending aorta at the highest point. Finally, the aortic cross-clamp is removed, multiple dearing maneuvers are undertaken, and eventually the patient is weaned off cardiopulmonary bypass. It is our practice to use transesophageal echocardiography (TEE) on all valve cases. At the latter part of the operation, prior to separation from cardiopulmonary bypass, the valve itself is inspected with TEE, as are the left atrium and ventricle to ensure that no air is present in those chambers. After separation from cardiopulmonary bypass, echo is used to confirm good valve function and for a final inspection of LV function.

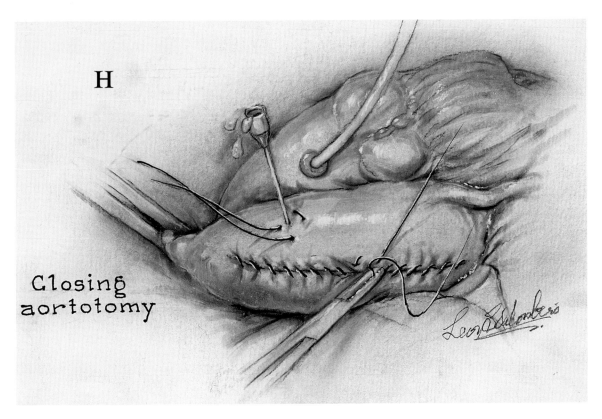

H

Closing
aortotomy

Chapter 14

The Ross Procedure

Duke E. Cameron, M.D.

Introduction

The Ross procedure (pulmonary valve autotransplant) is an ideal procedure for aortic valve replacement in selected patients. Advantages are excellent hemodynamics and durability, avoidance of anticoagulation, and a low incidence of thromboembolism and endocarditis. The autotransplanted valve may grow, making it the procedure of choice in infants and children.

A   After median sternotomy, institution of cardiopulmonary bypass, and cardioplegic arrest, a transverse aortotomy is made to inspect the aortic valve. A transverse pulmonary arteriotomy just proximal to the right pulmonary artery takeoff allows inspection of the pulmonary valve to ascertain its suitability for autotransplant.

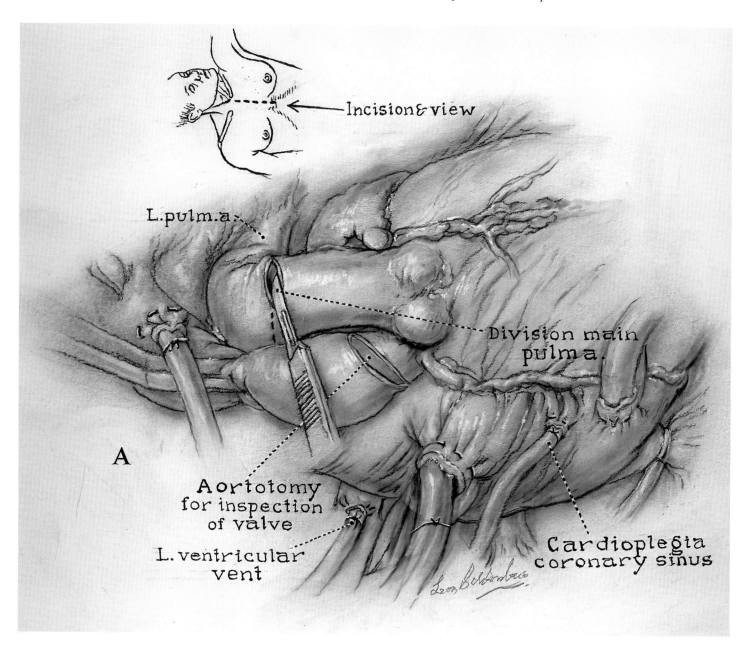

B The main pulmonary artery is completely transected and reflected anteriorly. A plane is dissected posteriorly between the pulmonary artery and the muscle of the right ventricular outflow tract and the left main coronary artery. The aortic valve leaflets have been excised.

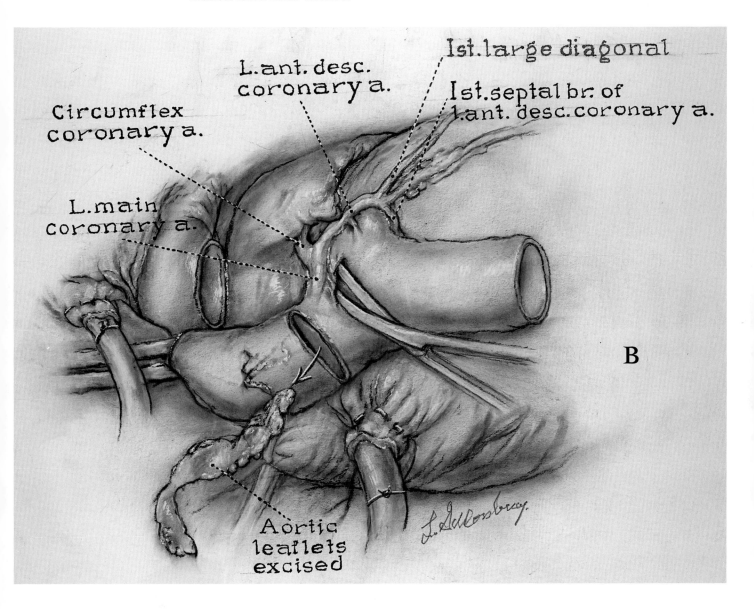

C Excision of the pulmonary root from the right ventricle is carried out with caution. A right-angled clamp is passed through the pulmonary valve and to a point 1 cm below the pulmonary valve. The anterior wall of the right ventricle is incised transversely.

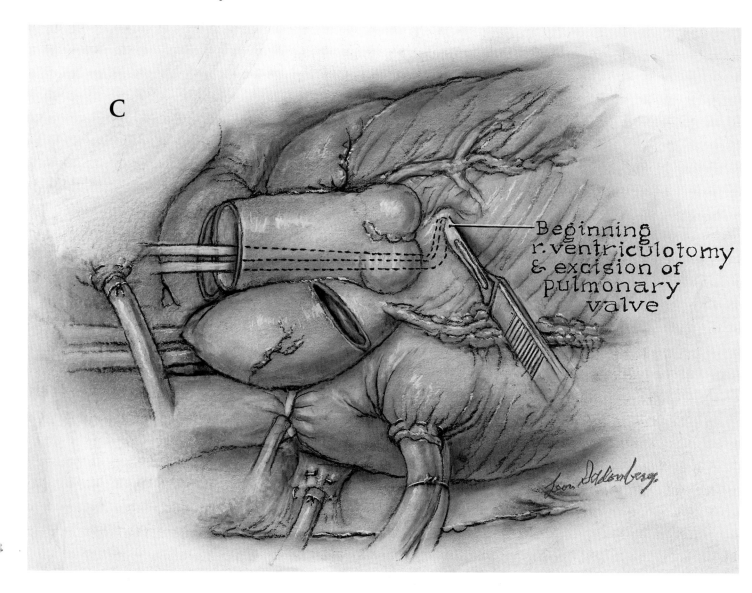

D The anterior right ventriculotomy is extended but should remain > 1 cm from the left anterior descending coronary artery (LAD). Posteriorly, the endocardium is scored with a scalpel, 1 cm proximal to the pulmonary valve.

E Excision of the pulmonary root is completed by dividing the muscle of the RVOT posteriorly in a tangential plane to avoid injury to the septal perforator of the LAD.

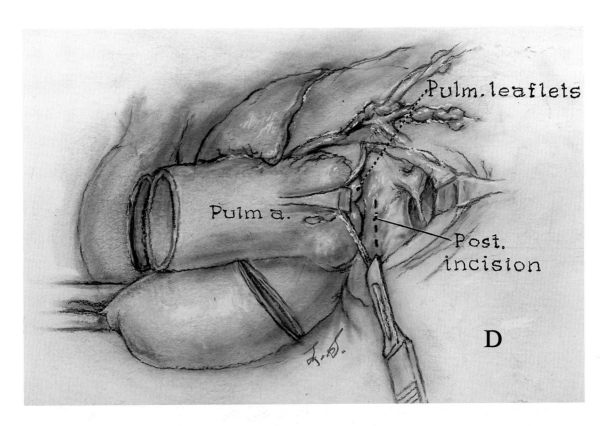

Pulm. leaflets

Pulm a.

Post.
incision

D

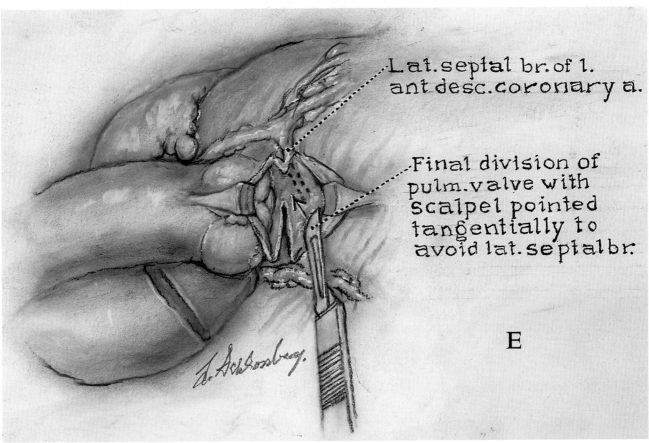

Lat. septal br. of 1.
ant. desc. coronary a.

Final division of
pulm. valve with
scalpel pointed
tangentially to
avoid lat. septal br.

E

F-G Pulmonary autograft can be anastomosed to the aortic annulus using continuous suture after placing 3 sutures at the nadir of each pulmonary sinus (shown) or alternatively by placing interrupted sutures. Sutures should include the annulus of pulmonary autograft to avoid late pseudoaneurysms.

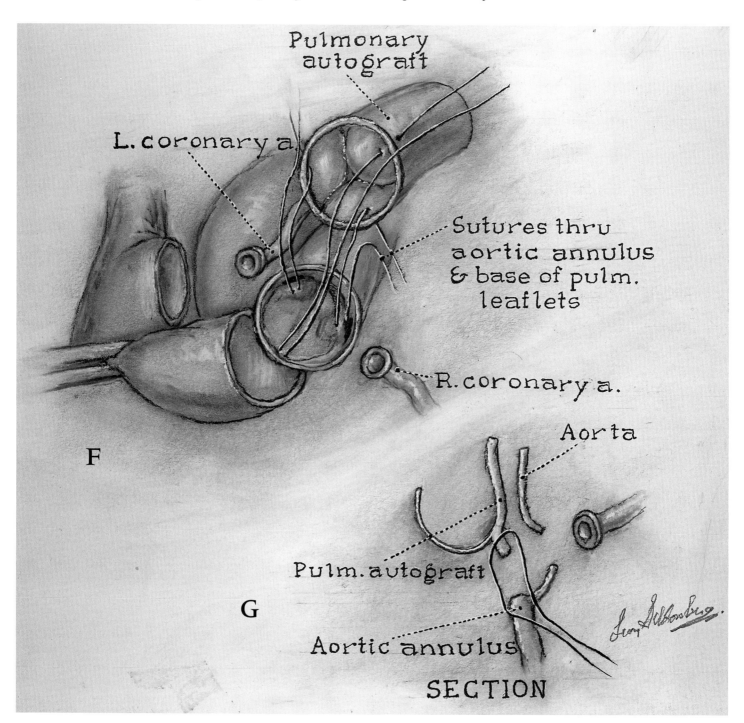

Pulmonary autograft

L. coronary a.

Sutures thru aortic annulus & base of pulm. leaflets

R. coronary a.

Aorta

F

Pulm. autograft

G

Aortic annulus

SECTION

H-I Coronary arteries are anastomosed to autograft sinuses with continuous sutures. A cryopreserved pulmonary valved homograft is sewn end-to-end to the distal native pulmonary artery. Exposure for this is better if done before the distal aorta anastomosis. After the aortic anastomosis, the proximal end of the pulmonary homograft is anastomosed to the RVOT with continuous suture. De-airing maneuvers and weaning from cardiopulmonary bypass are conducted in the standard manner.

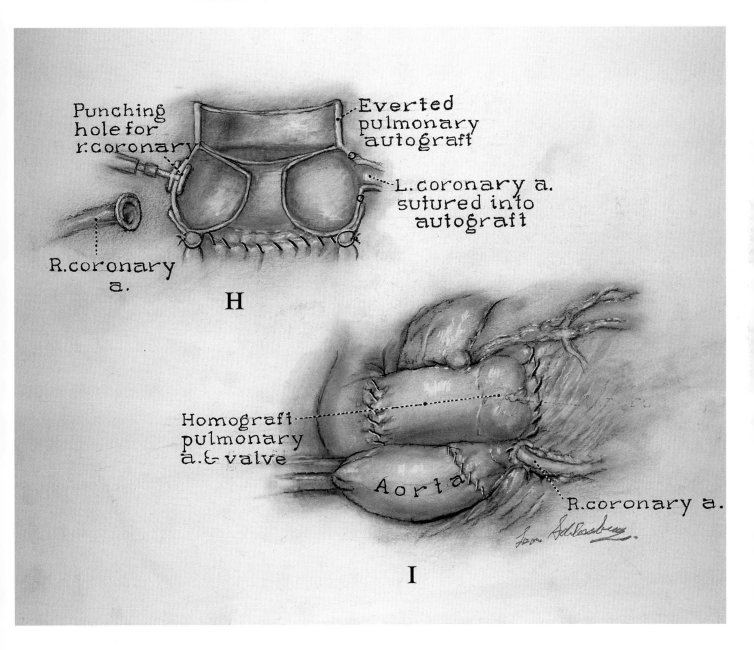

Punching hole for r.coronary

Everted pulmonary autograft

L.coronary a. sutured into autograft

R.coronary a.

H

Homograft pulmonary a. & valve

Aorta

R.coronary a.

I

Chapter 15

Supra-Coronary Aneurysm

Vincent L. Gott, M.D.

Introduction

Two different operative procedures are depicted in this section. The first supra-coronary aneurysm is a small post-stenotic aneurysm that is sometimes seen in patients undergoing aortic valve replacement. This type of aneurysm can be handled very easily by making a longitudinal aortotomy for the aortic valve replacement and then simply trimming the excess aortic wall from each side of the aortotomy, with closure as depicted. This procedure is suitable for post-stenotic aneurysms that are no larger than four centimeters in diameter.

For a larger supra-coronary aneurysm, a Dacron sleeve graft is required. It will be noted in several of the thoracic aortic procedures that the authors frequently reinforce anastomotic suture lines with a strip of Teflon felt. Felt reinforcement is particularly useful in patients with Marfan aneurysms or aneurysms secondary to aortic degenerative processes, and it does not add significant time to the procedure.

Small Supra-Coronary Aneurysm

A   A relatively small supra-coronary aneurysm with a longitudinal incision is shown; the excess aortic wall to be excised is indicated by stippling.

B   The aortic valve has been replaced with a bileaflet prosthesis, and the aortotomy is ready for closure.

C   Excess aortic wall is trimmed from both sides of the aortotomy.

D   The aortotomy is closed using two strips of Teflon felt with a running mattress suture.

E   The aortotomy closure is completed with a second over-and-over running suture.

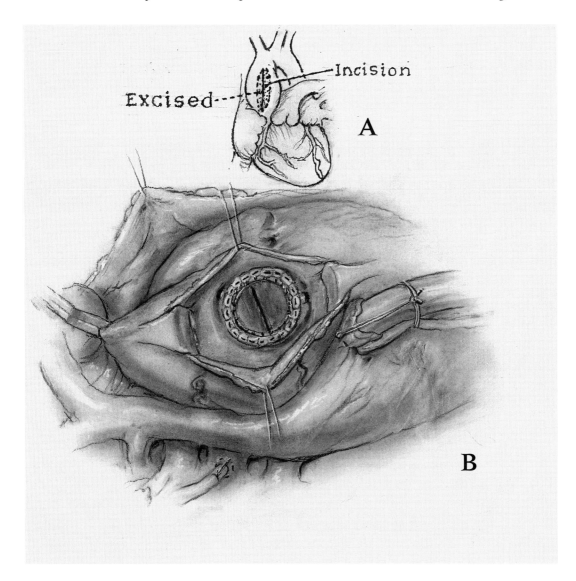

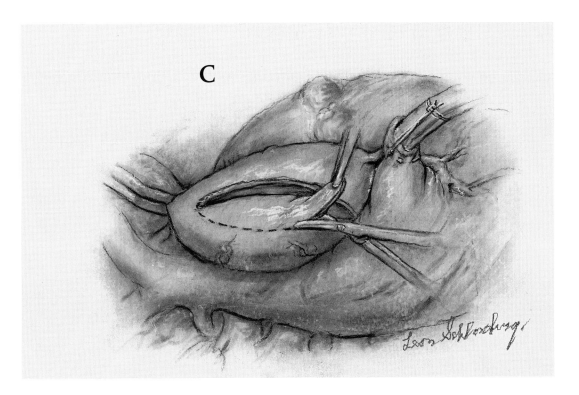

C

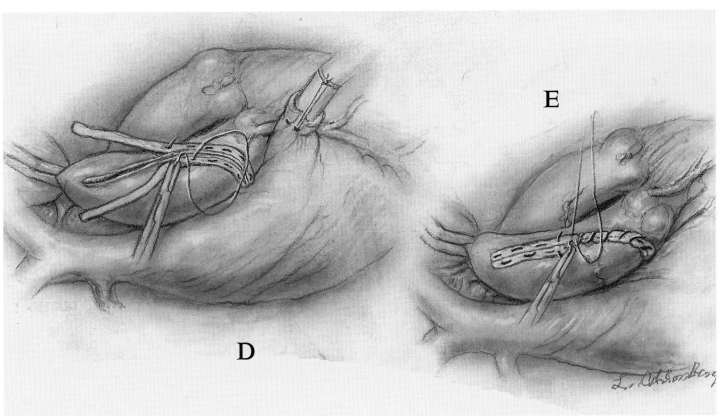

D

E

Large Supra-Coronary Aneurysm

A A sketch of a large supra-coronary aneurysm; the dotted lines indicate the site for aortic incisions.

B The patient is on cardiopulmonary bypass. The heart has been arrested and the aortic incision is being made.

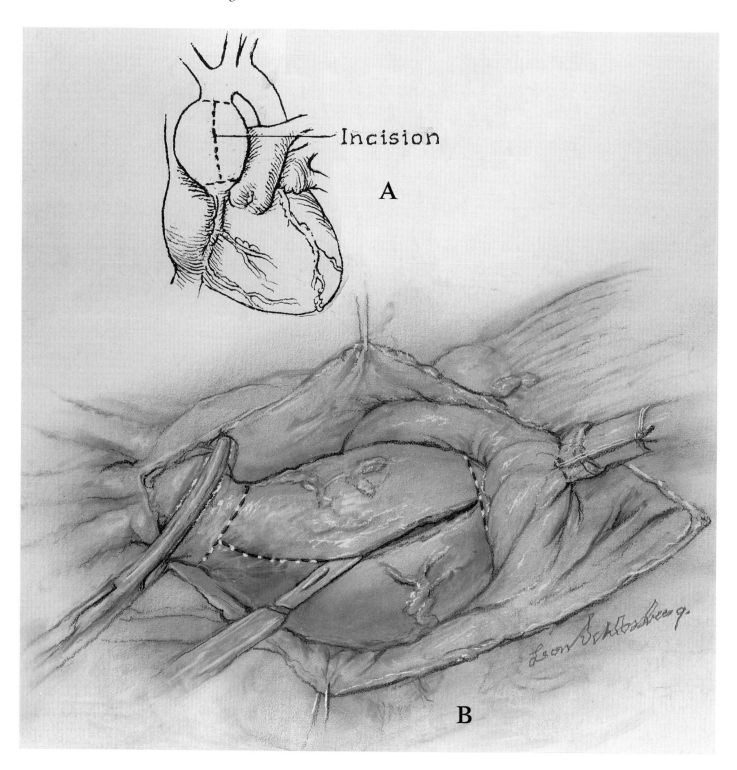

C   The proximal anastomosis is being constructed using a Dacron sleeve graft.

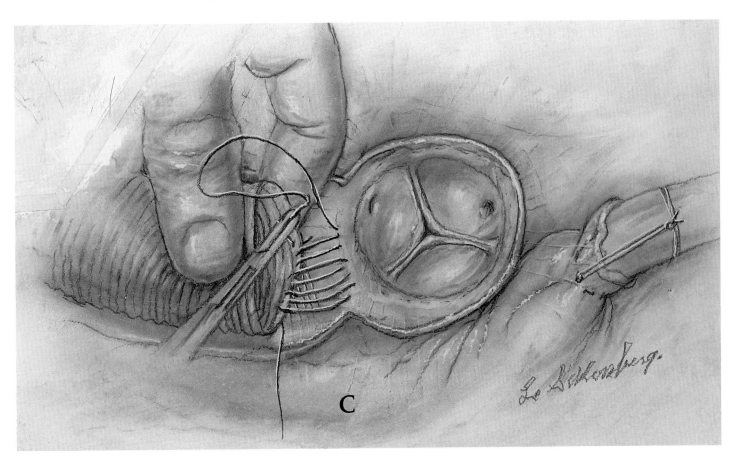

C

Large Supra-Coronary Aneurysm *continued*

D   The distal anastomosis is completed with a running polypropylene suture and a reinforcing strip of Teflon felt.

E   Excess wall of the aneurysm is being trimmed.

F   The aortic wall is loosely tacked over the graft to seal it off in the event of sternal infection. It is important that this suture line not be blood-tight.

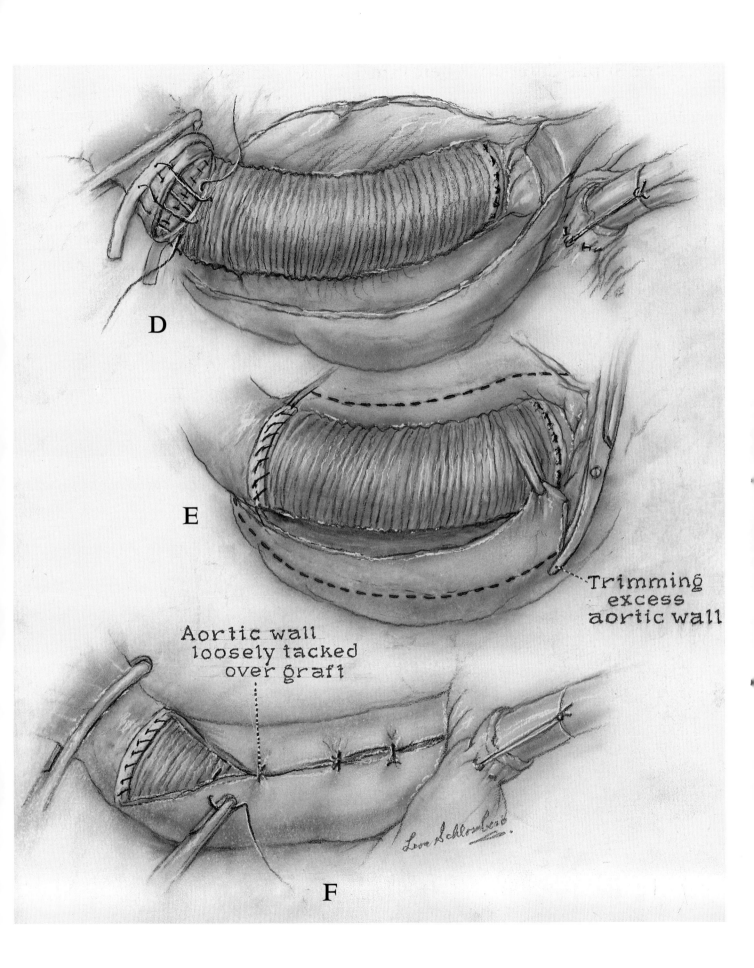

D

E

Trimming
excess
aortic wall

Aortic wall
loosely tacked
over graft

Leon Schlossberg.

F

Chapter 16

Operative Repair of DeBakey Type I(A) Aortic Dissection

Vincent L. Gott, M.D.

Introduction

Immediate operative repair is ordinarily required for an acute dissection of the ascending thoracic aorta, either DeBakey Type I or II or Stanford Type A. The procedure depicted can be used for chronic Type I dissection in that it employs an atraumatic vascular clamp across the distal ascending aorta. For many years, the author used an atraumatic vascular clamp in this position, even for acute Type I dissections, with good success. More recently, many surgeons operating on an acute dissection at this site do not place a clamp on the distal ascending aorta. When a vascular clamp is not used at this site, the patient should be cooled to at least 17° C and circulatory arrest employed while the distal anastomosis is completed.

A   The gross external appearance of the dissected ascending aorta is illustrated.

B   After cardioplegia, a longitudinal incision is made in the outer wall of the ascending aorta and, after exposing the false channel, the true channel is excised.

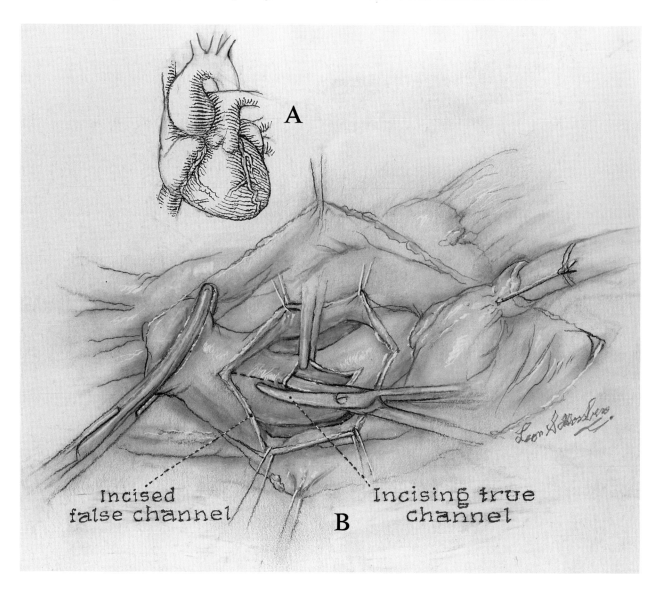

C   Again the author favors the use of Teflon felt strips to reinforce aortic suture lines. This is particularly helpful with the fragile aortic wall seen in acute Type I dissection. As shown in Figure C, strips of Teflon felt are sandwiched between the inner and outer aortic wall.

D   A running whipping stitch is used to oversew both the distal and the proximal ascending aorta.

E   Not infrequently, one or more of the aortic commissures becomes untethered during the dissection process; the commissures can be resuspended with a simple pledgeted suture as depicted.

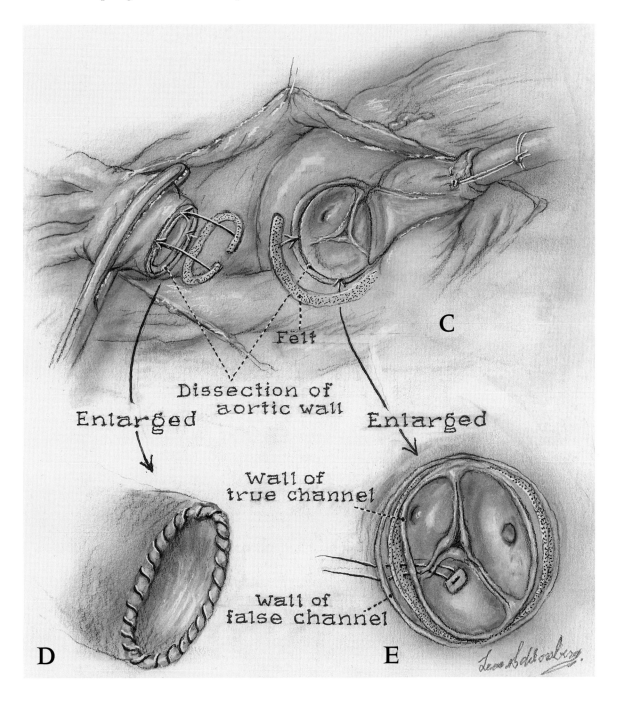

F Both the proximal and the distal ends of the ascending aorta have been prepared
for the placement of the graft.

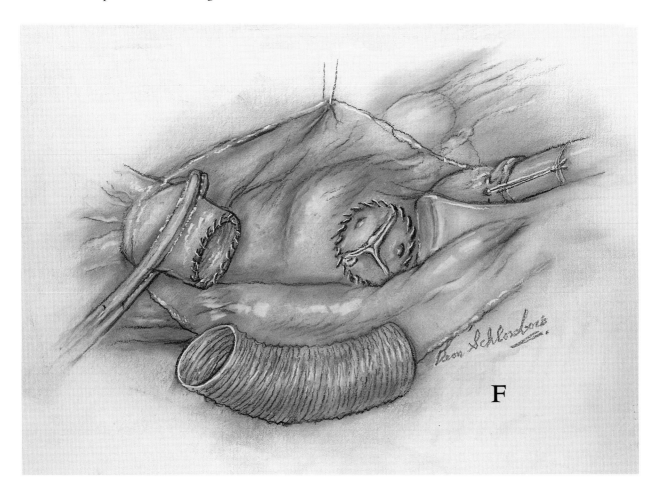

F

G The Dacron graft is in position and, in this case with a very friable aortic wall, an additional outer strip of Teflon felt is sued to reinforce the suture line.

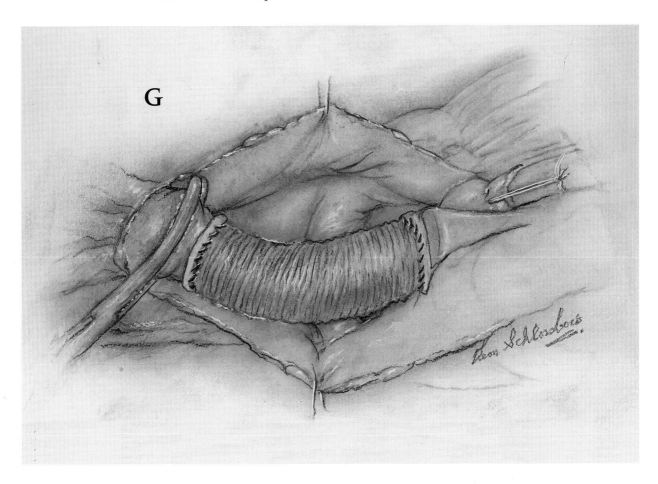

There are some excellent cardiovascular surgeons who pride themselves on never using Teflon felt to reinforce an aortic suture line. Even though these surgeons seem to have good operative results, this surgeon frequently reinforces an aortic anastomosis with a strip of Teflon felt. It adds very little time to the procedure, and although it may not always be necessary, it is rare that the surgeon has to place additional sutures in the anastomosis. Obviously, bleeding at a fairly inaccessible site in a suture line can be quite frustrating and can lead to increased morbidity and mortality.

Chapter 17

Classic Bentall Composite Graft Repair of a Marfan Aneurysm of the Ascending Aorta

Vincent L. Gott, M.D.

Introduction

The introduction of the composite graft repair for Marfan aneurysm of the ascending aorta by Mr. Hugh Bentall in 1968 (Bentall and DeBono, *Thorax* 23:338–9, 1968) markedly improved the extremely poor outlook for these patients. Before the availability of the Bentall procedure, Marfan patients with large aneurysms of the ascending aorta were rarely operated upon electively because a suitable operation was not available. Ordinarily, surgery was performed in these patients only with the development of acute aortic dissection or rupture. Between 1965 and 1976 the author operated on five Marfan patients with large aneurysms of the ascending aorta. Four of these patients came to the hospital with acute dissection and/or rupture; the fifth required urgent surgery because of severe congestive failure. Three of the five patients died during or immediately after the operative procedure. In September of 1976, we performed our first Bentall composite graft procedure for Marfan aneurysm of the ascending aorta. Over the next 22 years (through December 1998), Johns Hopkins surgeons performed performed aortic root replacement in 246 Marfan patients, with two hospital deaths. Both of these patients arrived in the operating room in a moribund condition with frank rupture of the aorta. Two hundred and twelve of the patients had elective repair and 34 had urgent repair primarily for dissection or rupture. Two hundred and twenty five patients underwent either the classic Bentall composite procedure described in this section or the newer modified Bentall procedure with coronary buttons. Twelve Marfan patients underwent aortic root replacement with a cryopreserved homograft root and nine Marfan patients underwent aortic root repair using the valve-sparing technique. In this section, the author describes the classic Bentall technique and, in the next section, the modified Bentall technique with coronary buttons. Dr. Duke Cameron describes aortic root replacement with a cryopreserved homograft root and the technique of aortic root repair with the valve-sparing procedure.

From the first Bentall procedure in 1976 through 1992, the author and his surgical colleagues favored the direct side-to-side coronary anastomosis illustrated in this section. More often than not in our early experience with the classic Bentall procedure, the coronary ostia had migrated cephalad adequately so that a direct side-to-side anastomosis could be carried out using a 4-0 polypropylene suture. If one or both of the coronary ostia were low, we would use a short vein graft or a 6.0 mm Dacron graft to bridge this segment.

In our initial experience with the classic Bentall procedure, we used the wall of the aortic aneurysm to construct a blood-tight enclosure of the composite graft. In one patient, we experienced tamponade between the encompassing aortic wrap and the Dacron graft; fortunately we were able to decompress this tamponade and obtain a successful outcome. Kouchoukos pointed out the importance of not creating a blood-tight wrap around the composite graft (Kouchoukos NT, Marshall WG, Wedige-Slecter TA: Eleven year experience with composite graft replacement of the ascending aorta and aortic valve. *J Thorac Cardiovasc Surg* 92:691, 1986), following which we simply tacked the residual aortic wall loosely over the graft to seal it off in the event of a sternal infection.

A   A standard sternal split incision is employed for this procedure.

B   Standard cardiopulmonary bypass is used, with body cooling to 27° C. Cardiac protection is ordinarily achieved with antegrade blood cardioplegia; retrograde blood cardioplegia is also used on occasion.

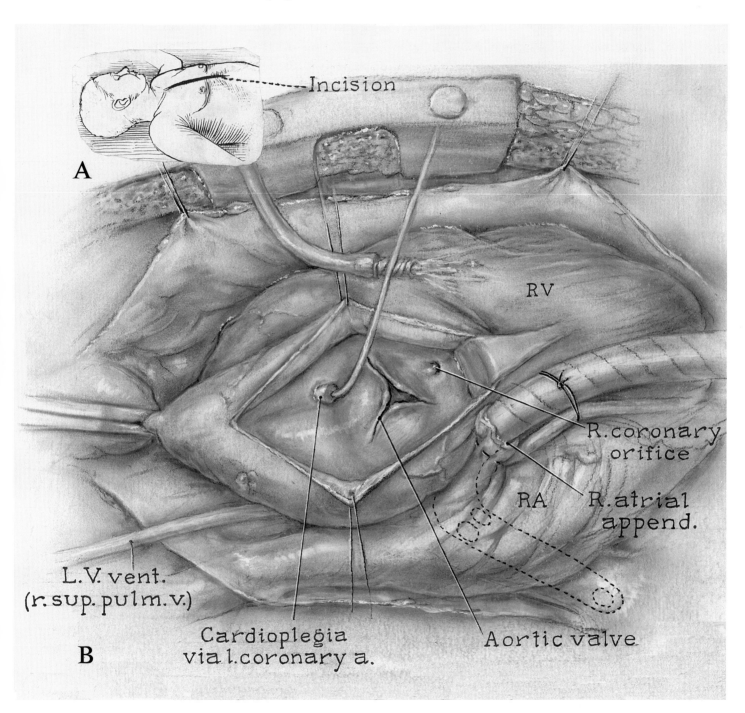

Artwork in this chapter originally appeared in Gott VL, et al: Ann Thorac Surg 52:38–45, 1991.

C-D The three leaflets have been excised.

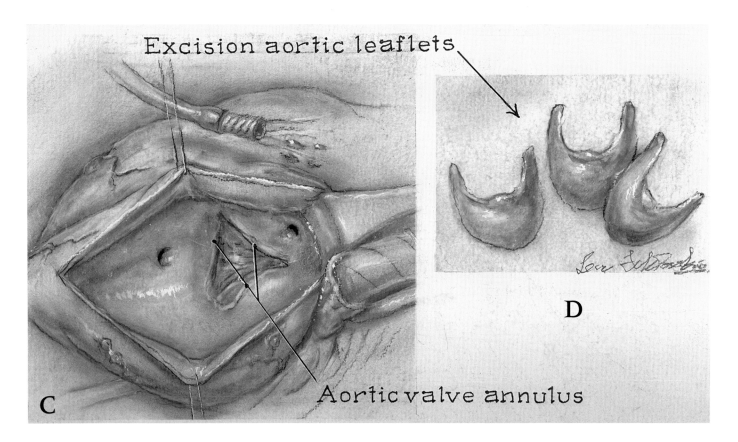

E Interrupted pledgeted 2-0 Tevdek sutures are placed in the annulus and then into the suture ring of the composite prosthesis. If the coronary arteries have migrated more than 12 mm from the annulus, we would use everting mattress sutures. If the coronary ostia are low-lying, then the placement of the mattress sutures beneath the annulus facilitates the direct anastomosis of the coronary ostia to the graft.

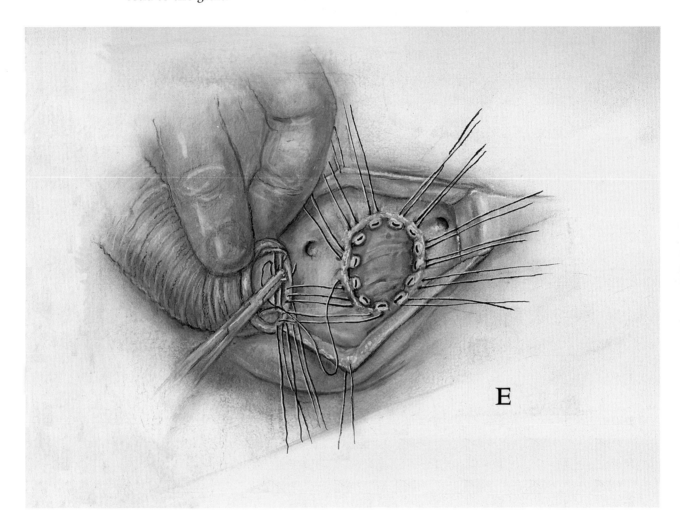

E

F All of the annular sutures have been tied, and the composite graft is in position.

G A running suture of a 4-0 polypropylene is used to construct a direct side-to-side anastomosis to the left coronary ostia.

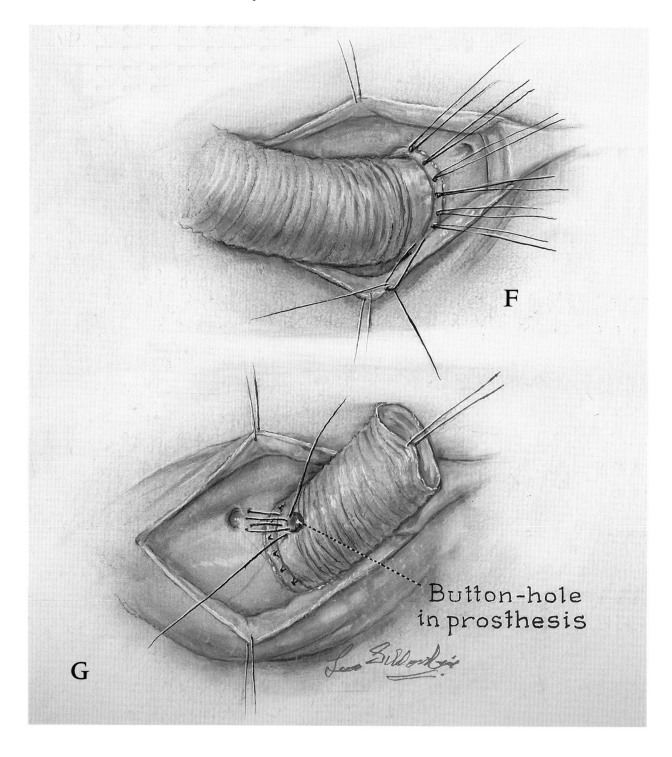

Button-hole
in prosthesis

F

G

H   A similar anastomosis is constructed to the right coronary ostia.

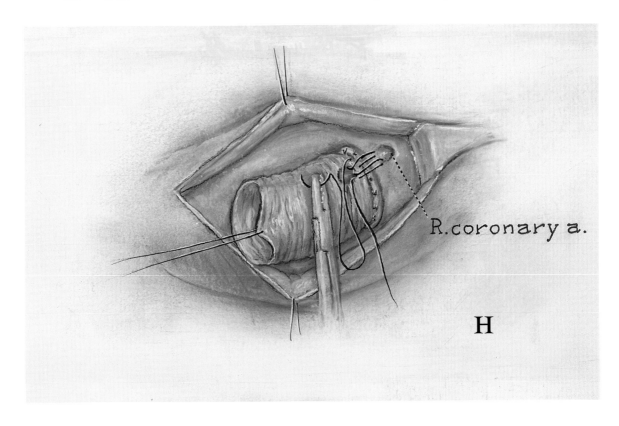

R. coronary a.

H

I   The distal ascending aorta is prepared for the distal anastomosis.

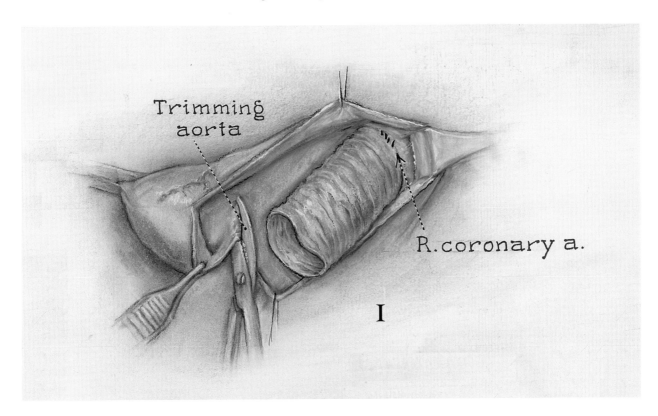

Trimming
aorta

R. coronary a.

I

J The distal anastomosis is completed with either a 3-0 or 4-0 polypropylene suture. The residual aneurysm wall is then trimmed and loosely tacked over the composite graft to protect it in the event of sternal infection.

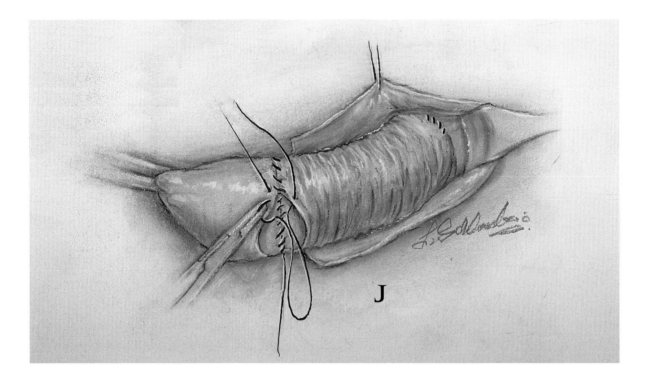

J

K The Cabrol interposed graft was used in a number of our early cases. We did discontinue the use of the Cabrol interposed graft in 1989 because of a kinking problem that developed in one of our patients. We did continue to use a 6.0 mm Dacron graft or saphenous vein segment in patients with low-lying coronary ostia. With the advent of the coronary button technique described in the next section, it has not been necessary to use any of these interposed coronary conduits in the Bentall operation.

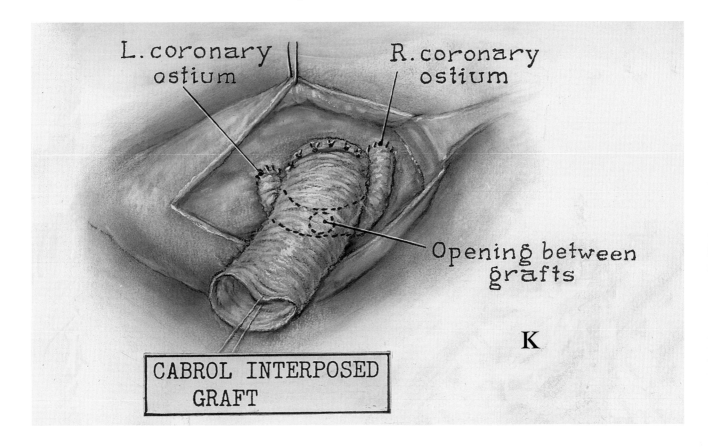

Chapter 18

Bentall Composite Graft for Marfan Aneurysm Using Coronary Buttons

Vincent L. Gott, M.D.

Introduction

The introduction of coronary buttons for the Bentall composite graft procedure in the early 1990's was a significant technical advance. Surgeons no longer had to worry about low-lying coronary ostia, which would require a Cabrol type procedure or an interposed vein graft. Another important advantage is that patients with smaller Marfan aneurysms can be operated upon without concern of achieving satisfactory coronary anastomoses. It has always been our policy to offer prophylactic repair of Marfan aneurysms when the diameter of the ascending aorta reaches 6.0 cm, even in patients who are asymptomatic. When the aortic root diameter is > 6.0 cm, aortic insufficiency usually develops and the patients become symptomatic. The majority of patients though with an aortic root of 6.0 cm have competent aortic valves and are asymptomatic. It is rare for a Marfan aneurysm of 6.0 cm or less to dissect, although we have seen dissection at 5.0 to 5.5 cm. With the availability of the coronary button technique, we now frequently recommend surgery when the aortic root reaches 5.5 cm; if there is a family history of dissection, we recommend operative intervention with a diameter of 5.0 cm.

In this section we depict our technique of aortic root resection using the Bentall composite graft with coronary buttons. The technique of cardiopulmonary bypass and antegrade blood cardioplegia is the same as in the previous section.

A   A standard sternal split incision is used.

B   This sketch shows a typical Marfan aneurysm of the ascending aorta that is 7.0 cm in diameter.

C   The ascending aorta has been opened and the aortic valve is being excised.

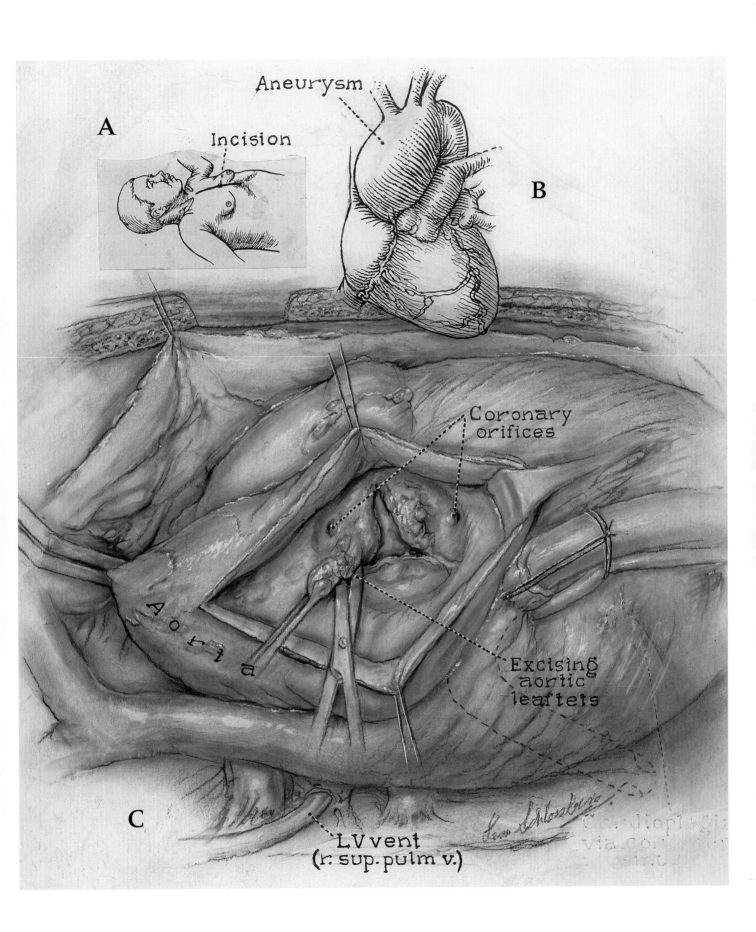

A

Incision

Aneurysm

B

Coronary
orifices

Aorta

Excising
aortic
leaflets

C

LV vent
(r. sup. pulm v.)

D   The surgeon is creating a button of aortic wall around the right coronary ostia.

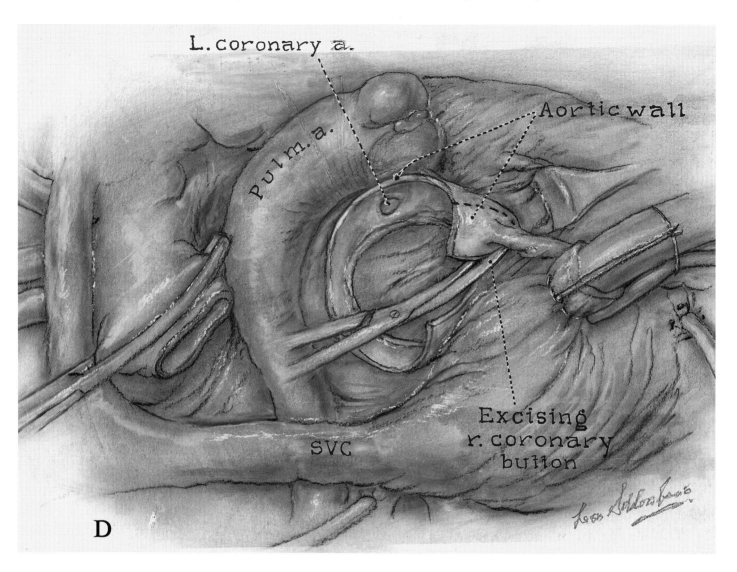

E   Interrupted pledgeted mattress sutures of 2-0 Tevdek have been placed in the annulus and are being passed through the sewing ring of the composite graft. The two coronary buttons have been prepared for anastomosis to the graft.

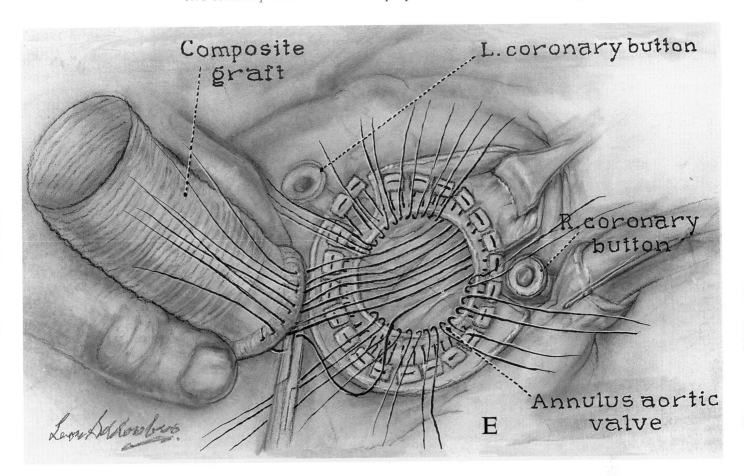

Composite graft

L. coronary button

R. coronary button

Annulus aortic valve

E

F   Both coronary vessels have been sutured to the base of the Dacron graft using Teflon felt reinforcement washers. The distal anastomosis is being constructed with a reinforcing strip of Teflon felt.

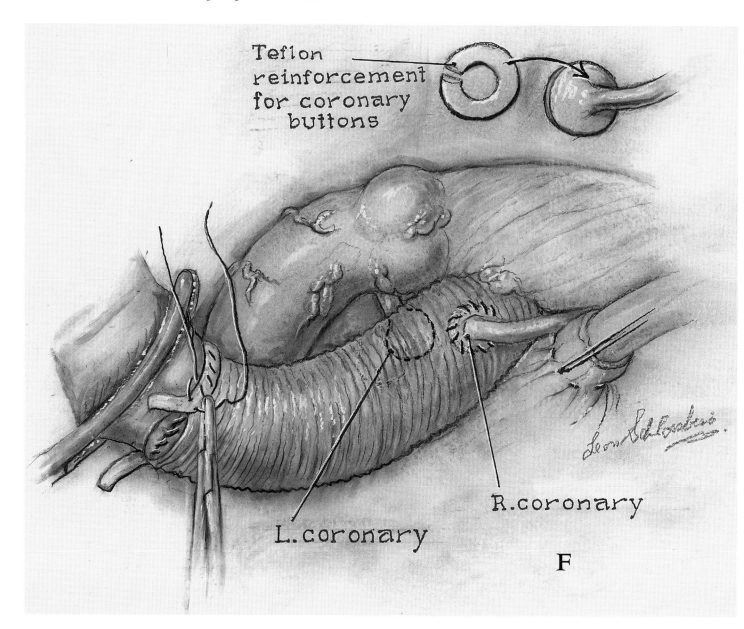

Chapter 19

Homograft Aortic Root Replacement

Duke E. Cameron, M.D.

Introduction

Aortic root replacement with a homograft is indicated for prosthetic endocarditis or in some situations when a bioprosthesis is preferred over a mechanical prosthesis, especially in children or adults with a small aortic root. Our technique is similar to that for aortic root replacement using a composite graft. Moderately hypothermic cardiopulmonary bypass is used (28–30° C) and standard cardioplegic techniques employed. Venting is usually via the right superior pulmonary vein.

A The aortic root is excised and the coronary arteries are mobilized. Everting horizontal mattress sutures are placed around the aortic annulus and then through the base of the homograft. In the setting of active endocarditis, no Teflon felt is used, and monofilament nonabsorbable sutures are preferred. We have found it useful to reinforce the proximal homograft suture line with strips of pericardium (in endocarditis) or Teflon felt (noninfected cases) for homeostasis. The coronary artery implants are performed with continuous suture, the left coronary first and then the right coronary.

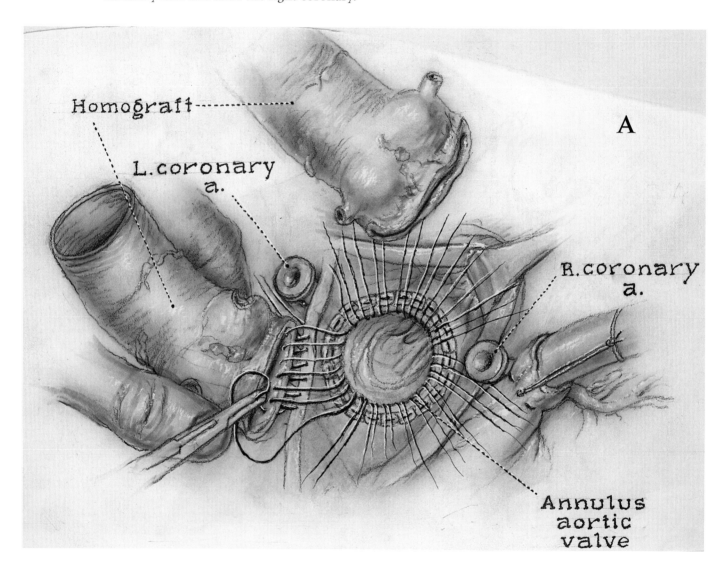

B   The distal homograft-to-aorta suture line is completed with continuous monofilament nonabsorbable suture.

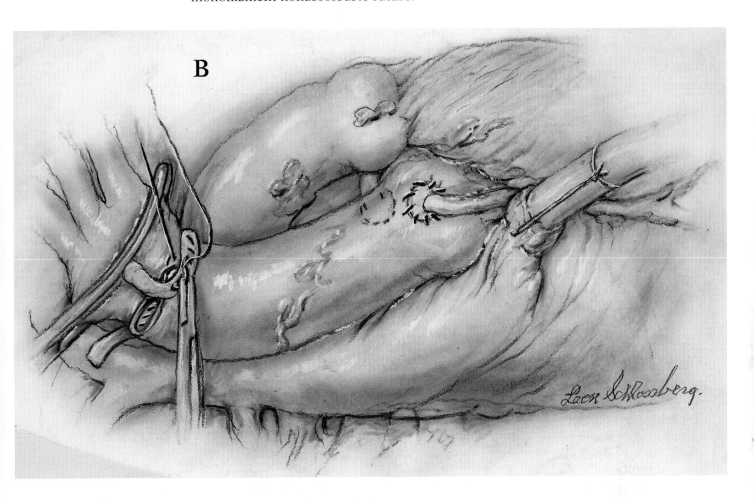

B

Chapter 20

Valve-sparing Aortic Root Replacement

Duke E. Cameron, M.D.

Introduction

Replacement of the aneurysmal ascending aorta from the annulus to the innominate artery can eliminate the risk of aneurysm rupture or dissection. In some cases, the aortic valve can be preserved, thus avoiding the complications of valve prostheses and anticoagulation. Cannulation, venting, cardioplegic arrest, and cardiopulmonary bypass are similar to that used for conventional aortic root surgery.

A   We have found it advantageous for exposure of the root to cannulate the cavae separately, placing the superior vena cava cannula through the right atrial appendage; this retracts the appendage away from the aortic root.

B   The aortic root is excised, leaving a 3–4 mm margin of aortic sinus tissue along the aortic annulus. The coronary arteries are widely mobilized.

C   A felt strip can be placed to reduce the aortic annulus to address aorto-annular ectasia. In our current practice, a purse-string suture is placed through the nadir of each sinus tongue of the graft to stabilize the annular diameter.

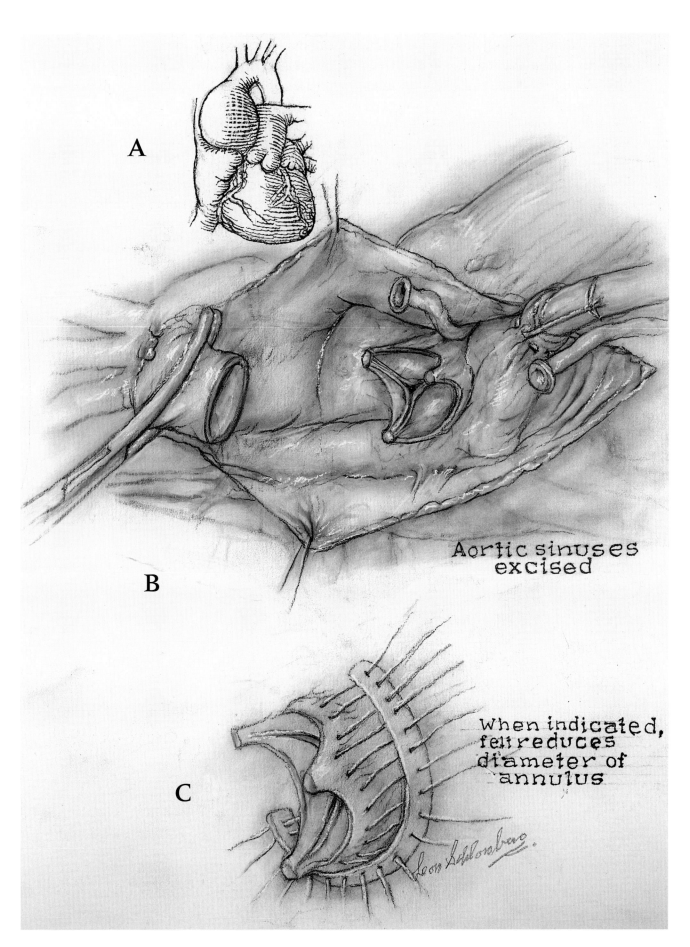

A

B

Aortic sinuses
excised

C

When indicated,
felt reduces
diameter of
annulus

Leon Schlossberg.

D A Dacron graft having a diameter of the sinotubular junction that optimizes leaflet coaptation (usually 28–30 mm in an adult) is then sewn to the aortic annulus. Three horizontal mattress sutures of 4-0 polypropylene are placed from inside the graft at the top of the vertical incisions made for each of the commissures. The height of these incisions is approximately ⅔ of the diameter of the graft. These sutures are passed through the aorta at the top of the commissures. Then one arm of each suture is run continuously through the aortic annulus and the graft to seat the graft to the aortic annulus. Felt-strip reinforcement of this suture line facilitates hemostasis.

E Holes are cut in the Dacron graft opposite the coronary arteries which are encircled with Teflon-felt "lifesaver" pledgets and anastomosed to the graft with continuous 4-0 polypropylene. The remaining portions of the operation are conducted in a manner similar to other aortic root procedures.

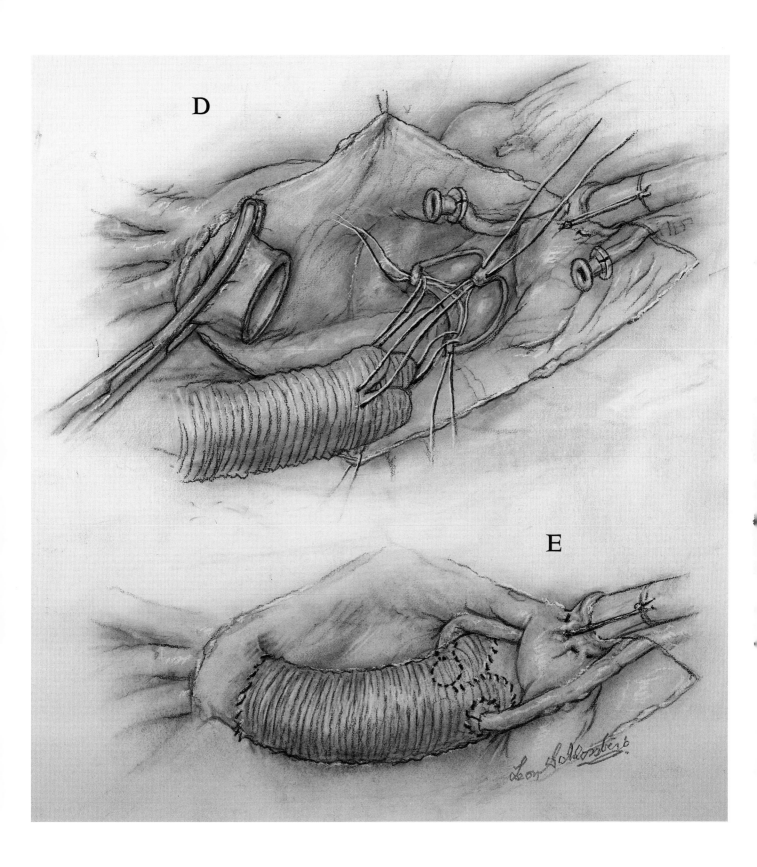

D

E

Chapter 21

Classic Aortic Arch Replacement with Aortic Root Replacement Using a Composite Graft

Duke E. Cameron, M.D.

Introduction

Large aneurysms involving the ascending aorta and arch are usually handled by replacement of the ascending aorta with a composite graft and replacement of the arch with a Dacron graft.

A   Median sternotomy is employed.

B   A large aneurysm of the ascending aorta may make femoral arterial cannulation advisable, but alternatively the aneurysm can be cannulated directly for initial cardiopulmonary bypass and cooling.

C   While cooling for hypothermic circulatory arrest for arch replacement, the ascending aorta is clamped and resected, the coronary arteries mobilized, and the aortic valve excised. The aortic annulus is rimmed with horizontal mattress sutures of pledgeted braided polyester suture. These sutures are passed through the sewing cuff of the composite graft, which is lowered into place and the sutures tied and cut. Holes are cut in the graft opposite the coronary arteries, which are anastomosed to the ascending aortic graft with continuous polypropylene suture.

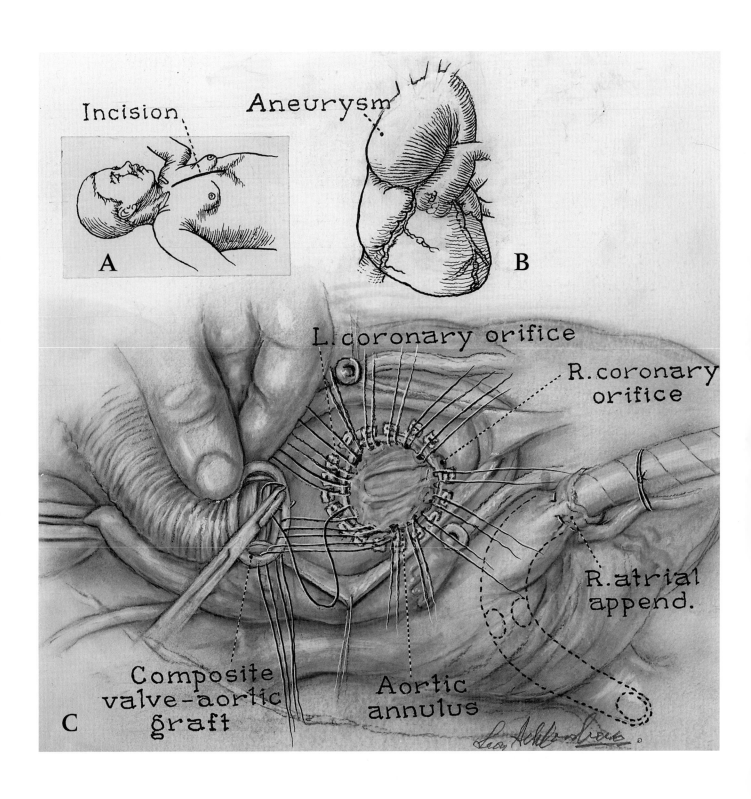

Incision

Aneurysm

A

B

L. coronary orifice

R. coronary orifice

Composite
valve-aortic
graft

Aortic
annulus

R. atrial
append.

C

Artwork in this chapter originally appeared in Baumgartner WA, et al: The Johns Hopkins Manual of Cardiac Surgical Care. St. Louis, Mosby, 1994.

D   Circulatory arrest is induced and the patient placed in Trendelenburg position.

E   Under circulatory arrest, the transverse arch is incised. A Dacron graft having the diameter of of the proximal descending aorta is selected.

F   A hole is cut in the side of the graft for the "island" of neck vessels.

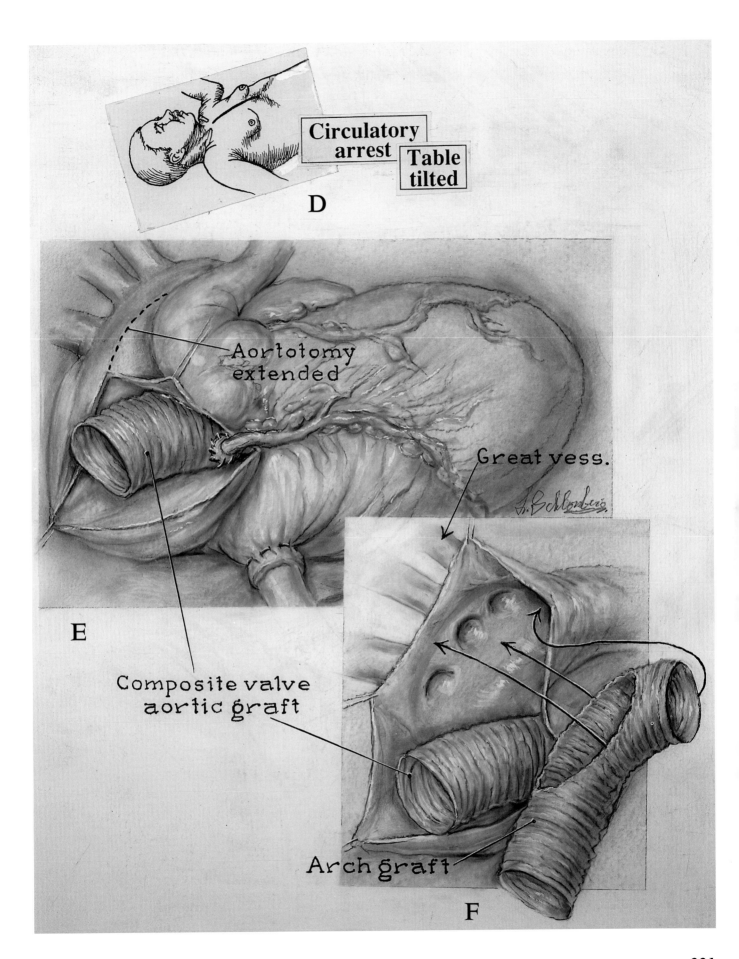

Circulatory arrest

Table tilted

D

Aortotomy extended

Great vess.

E

Composite valve aortic graft

Arch graft

F

G After the distal anastomosis is completed (which is sometimes facilitated by inverting the graft into the descending aorta), the side-to-side anastomosis of the arch vessel island to the side hole of the graft is performed.

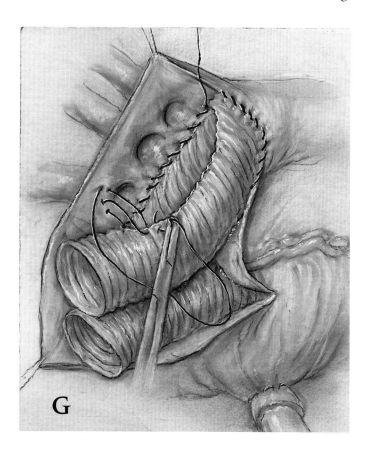

G

H The ascending aortic graft is anastomosed to the transverse arch graft end-to-end. This can usually be done with a cross-clamp applied to the proximal end of the arch graft to minimize circulatory arrest time.

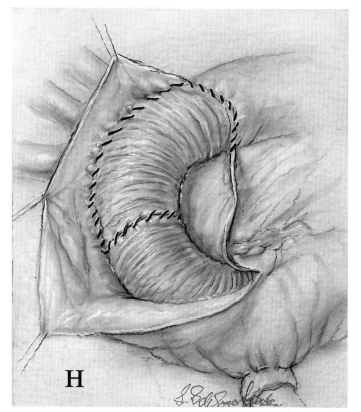

H

I   When the arch dilatation is mild, a hemi-arch replacement will suffice and will shorten circulatory arrest time.

J   A beveled Dacron graft is sewn to the undersurface of the arch.

K   The anastomoses are completed.

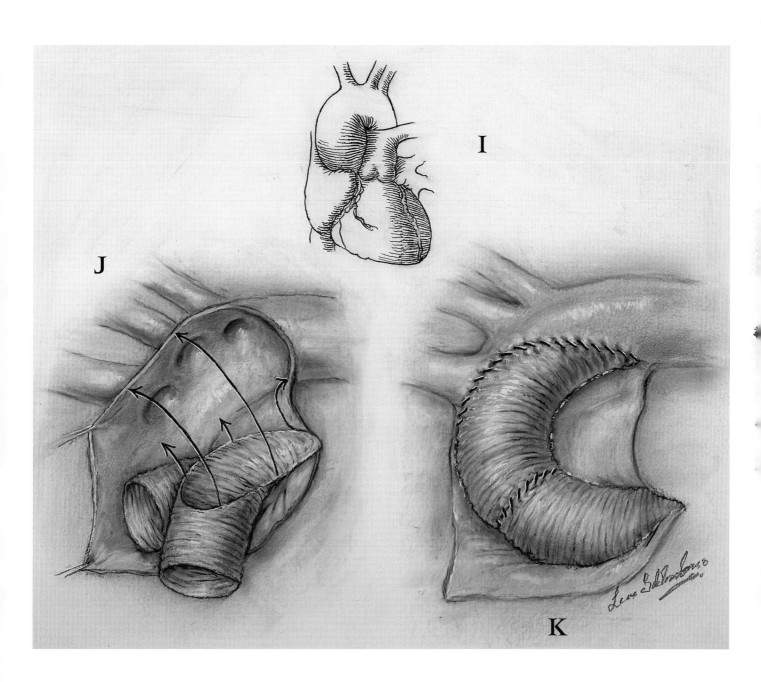

L The extended hypothermic circulatory arrest times sometimes necessary in complex arch reconstruction can be made safer by retrograde cerebral perfusion. The superior vena cava cannula can be used to provide retrograde perfusion of oxygenated blood to the brain and maintain cerebral hypothermia.

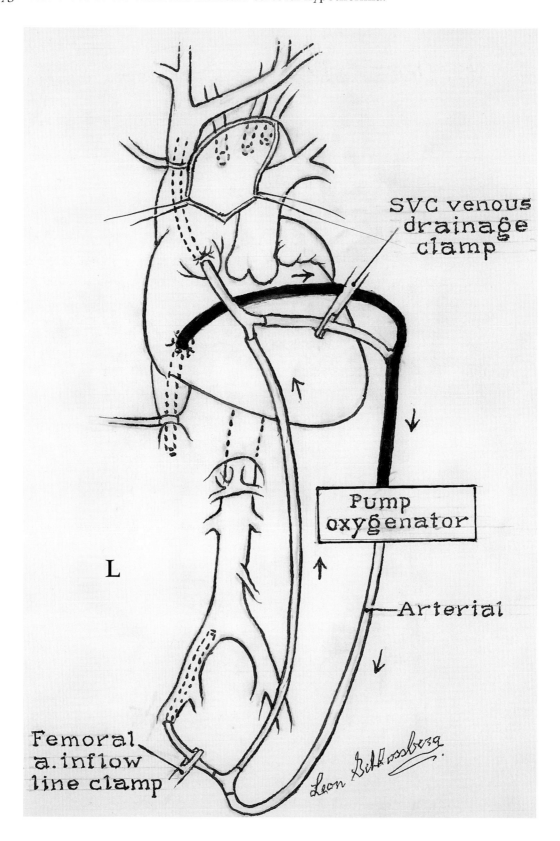

Chapter 22

The Elephant Trunk Procedure

Duke E. Cameron, M.D.

Introduction

Replacement of the ascending aorta, arch, and descending aorta for aneurysmal disease is facilitated by a staged approach using the "elephant trunk" procedure. The ascending aorta and arch are replaced first with a Dacron graft. The distal end of the graft lies within the proximal descending thoracic aorta like an elephant trunk; it will facilitate the proximal anastomosis for the later descending aortic replacement.

A Median sternotomy is used with femoral arterial and bicaval venous cannulation. A coronary sinus catheter can be used for intermittent retrograde coronary sinus perfusion. A vent is placed in the right superior pulmonary vein. The aortic arch is dissected and the vagus nerve freed from the transverse arch to avoid injury to the recurrent laryngeal nerve. After cross-clamping and cardioplegic arrest of the heart, circulatory arrest is induced and the ascending aorta incised. The incision is taken into the anterior surface of the mid-arch.

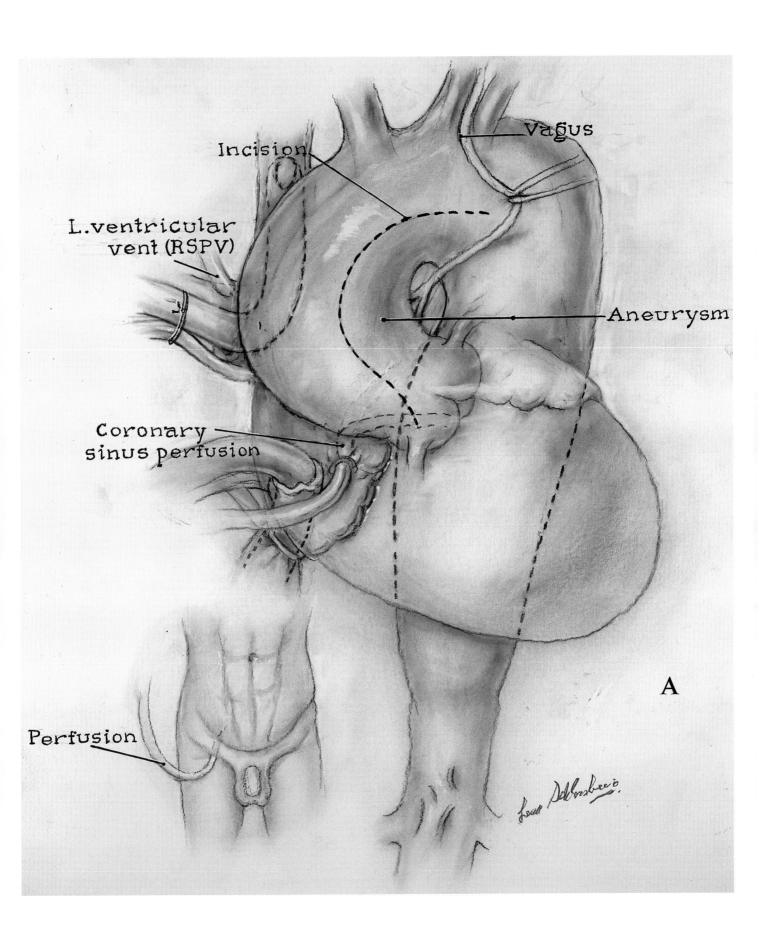

B A tag suture is placed on the end of a woven Dacron graft.

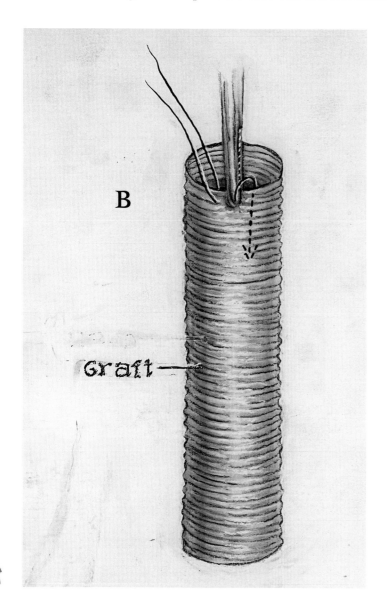

Graft

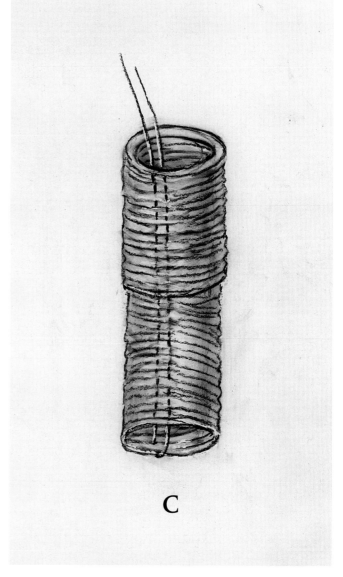

C The graft is intussuscepted as shown. The distal segment of the graft that extends beyond the distal arch anastomosis should be no longer than 6 cm in length to avoid occlusion of important intercostal vessels

.D The graft is placed into the descending thoracic aorta. The distal anastomosis is performed within the aorta to the folded edge of the graft with continuous polypropylene suture.

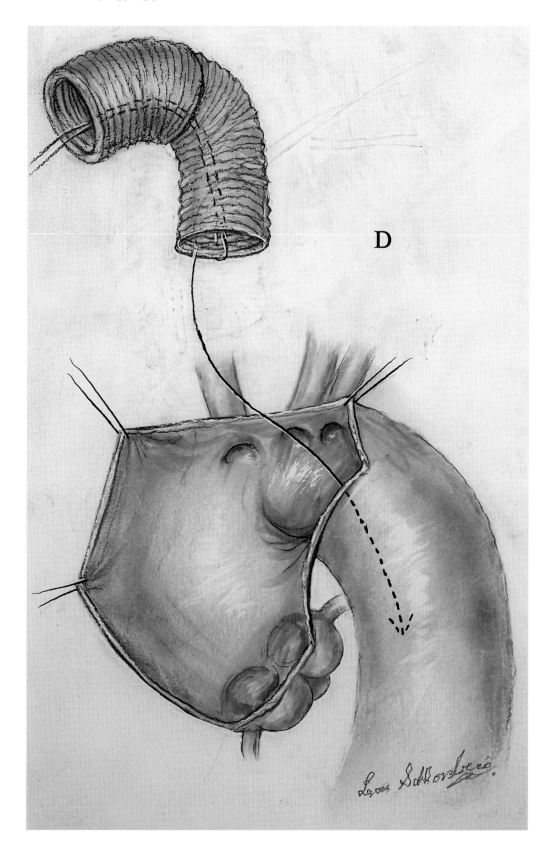

D

E   The stay suture is pulled back, retracting the graft into the arch and ascending aorta.

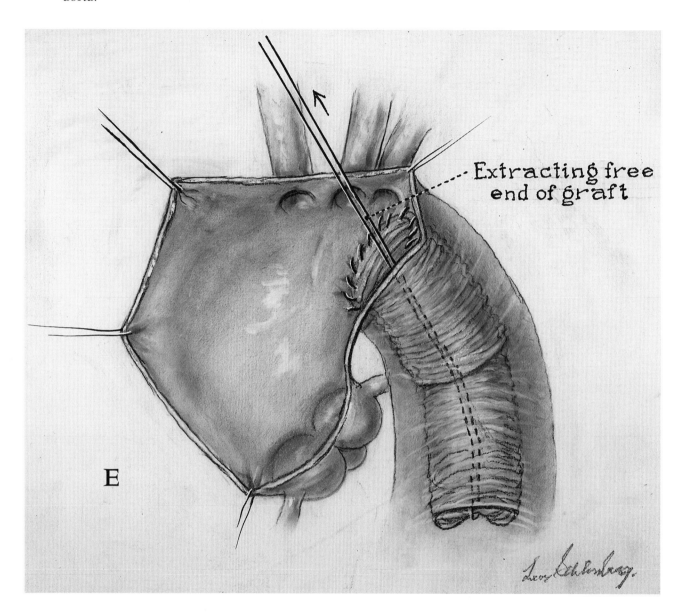

E

F   A large side hole is cut in the cephalad aspect of the graft, which is anastomosed to an island of arch vessels with continuous suture. Replacement of the ascending aorta or aortic root is performed using techniques described elsewhere in this section.

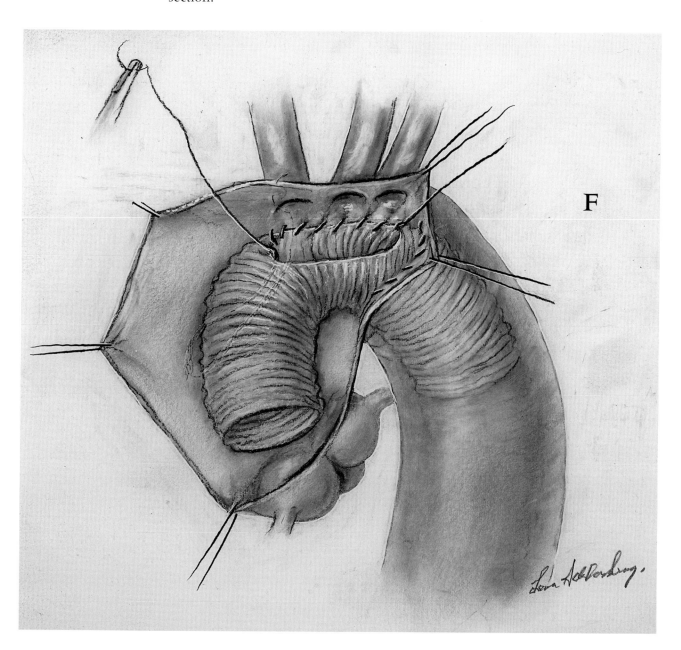

F

Chapter 23

Replacement of the Distal Aortic Arch and Proximal Descending Thoracic Aorta

J. Mark Redmond, M.D.

Introduction

Distal aortic arch and proximal descending thoracic aortic procedures are usually performed through a left posterolateral thoracotomy incision; they require full cardiopulmonary bypass with circulatory arrest if it is not possible to place a clamp between the left common carotid artery without compromising the proximal anastomosis. In this section, replacement of this portion of the aorta is described for a distal aortic arch aneurysm associated with an anomalous origin of the right subclavian artery from the proximal descending thoracic aorta. The proximal portion of the right subclavian artery was also aneurysmal, causing compression of the esophagus for the patient. In preparation for repair, the patient had undergone a right common carotid to right subclavian artery bypass, with ligation of the right subclavian artery proximal to the anastomosis, through a right supraclavicular incision.

The second stage of the operation is performed through a left posterolateral thoracotomy incision. A spinal drain is placed for augmented cord protection on the day prior to surgery. Following induction of general anesthesia, a double lumen endothracheal tube is placed; satisfactory position and function are confirmed using a flexible bronchoscope. After placement of bilateral radial arterial lines along with central venous and pulmonary arterial catheters, the patient is positioned for left thoracotomy in standard fashion, though the hips are rotated more anteriorly than usual, to provide access to both groin regions. The operating table is flexed to the desired extent. The latissimus dorsi muscle is divided and, while much of the serratus anterior muscle can be spared, its attachments to the fourth, fifth, and sixth ribs are transected, using electrocautery. The left pleural space is entered either through the fourth or the fifth intercostal space, depending on the distal extent of the descending thoracic aorta to be replaced. It is possible to reach the distal aorta at the level of the diaphragm through the fifth and certainly through the sixth intercostal spaces. It may be necessary to notch the rib above for additional access to the aortic arch when a lower intercostal space is chosen.

Following placement of a rib-spreading retractor or other external retractor system, the deflated left lung is reflected anteromedially, and the aortic arch and descending thoracic aorta are dissected. During dissection, the phrenic and vagus nerves together with the recurrent laryngeal nerve are usually visualized and vessel loops placed around each nerve pedicle for later retraction during performance of the proximal anastomosis. Simultaneously, a groin incision is made, and dissection of the sapheno-femoral venous junction together with the left common femoral artery is undertaken. Heparin is administered and preparations for cannulation are made.

A   Total cardiopulmonary bypass and hypothermic circulatory arrest are necessary for repair. A purse-string suture is placed at the saphenofemoral junction, and the right femoral vein is cannulated using a 28 French venous cannula, which is passed through the inferior vena cava to the right atrium. Its position in the mid-portion of the right atrium is confirmed by transesophageal echocardiography. Having divided the inferior pulmonary ligament, the inferior pulmonary vein is dissected. A purse-string suture is placed, and an angle venous cannula, usually of 24F caliber, is positioned in the left atrium. Meanwhile, an 8-mm Dacron tube graft has been sutured end-to-side to the left common femoral artery using the running 5-0 Prolene suture. The Dacron graft is cannulated with a short arterial cannula and secured. A second line is "Y'd" off the arterial line for later reperfusion of the proximal portion of the aortic graft following circulatory arrest. Cardiopulmonary bypass is initiated, and, once adequate decompression of the left ventricle is confirmed by inspection and by transesophageal echocardiography, cooling is begun. Adjustment of the right atrial cannula is occasionally required to ensure satisfactory venous drainage. The arrangement of the cardiopulmonary bypass circuit and the aortic and venous cannulae are depicted in this diagram. Cooling for 40 minutes is generally undertaken with a final arterial inflow temperature of 13° C. The esophageal temperature is usually in the 14° C to 16° C range with bladder or rectal temperature of 18° at the end of the cooling phase. Before circulatory arrest is initiated, ice packs are placed on the head and steroids administered intravenously. The field is flooded with carbon dioxide gas and delivered through tubing sutured to the skin edge at one end of the incision to facilitate de-airing later. The patient is then placed in Trendelenburg position.

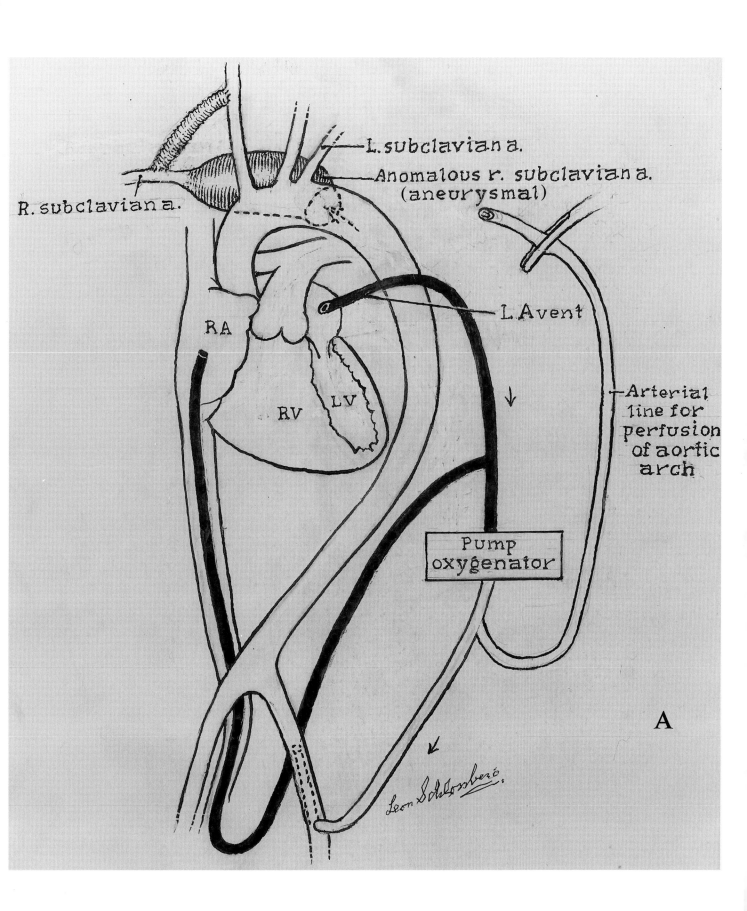

L. subclavian a.

Anomalous r. subclavian a.
(aneurysmal)

R. subclavian a.

L. A vent

RA

RV   LV

Arterial
line for
perfusion
of aortic
arch

Pump
oxygenator

A

Leon Schlossberg

B   The descending thoracic aorta is cross-clamped at the level of T5 and circulatory arrest is begun. Perfusion below the cross-clamp is continued and monitored by an arterial line placed in the left or right femoral artery. The aneurysmal portion of the descending thoracic aorta is opened and the incision continued into the distal aortic arch. Stay sutures are placed in the aortic wall, and the highest of the intercostal vessels are oversewn from within the aorta if they have not been clipped externally during cooling. The aorta is transected at the level of the left subclavian artery. Care is taken to avoid injury to the esophagus, which is in close proximity. A portion of the aneurysmal distal aortic arch and proximal descending aorta together with the proximal portion of the aneurysmal right subclavian artery is resected and sent for pathologic evaluation.

C   A strip of reinforcing Teflon felt is sutured circumferentially to the distal aortic arch. A previously selected tube graft of Hemashield of appropriate caliber, to which has been anastomosed an 8-mm Hemashield tube graft in end-to-side fashion, is now brought into the field. The side arm will serve both for reperfusion to the upper body after circulatory arrest and, if necessary, for an end-to-end anastomosis to the left subclavian artery should the origin of the left subclavian artery be involved in the aneurysmal process. An end-to-end anastomosis between the distal arch and the tube graft is performed using a running 3-0 monofilament suture.

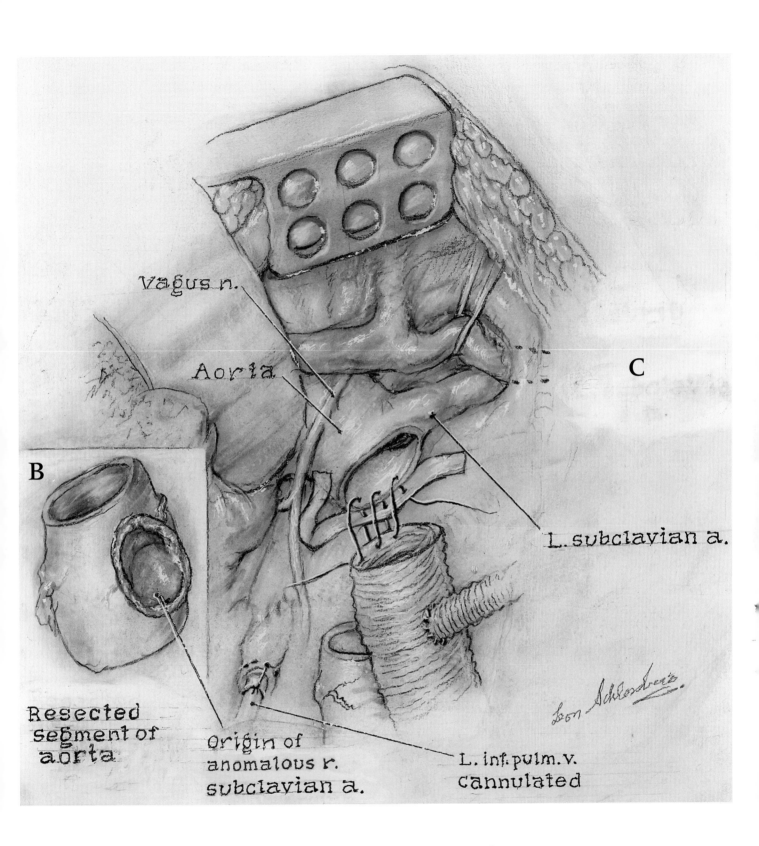

Vagus n.

Aorta

B

Resected
segment of
aorta

Origin of
anomalous r.
subclavian a.

C

L. subclavian a.

L. inf. pulm. v.
cannulated

D Once the anastomosis is complete, the 8-mm side arm is cannulated and perfusion of the aortic arch is gradually resumed to aid in de-airing the aortic arch and the graft, which is then clamped distal to the side arm. Cardiopulmonary bypass is reinstituted and the patient rewarmed after hemostasis is confirmed along the proximal suture line.

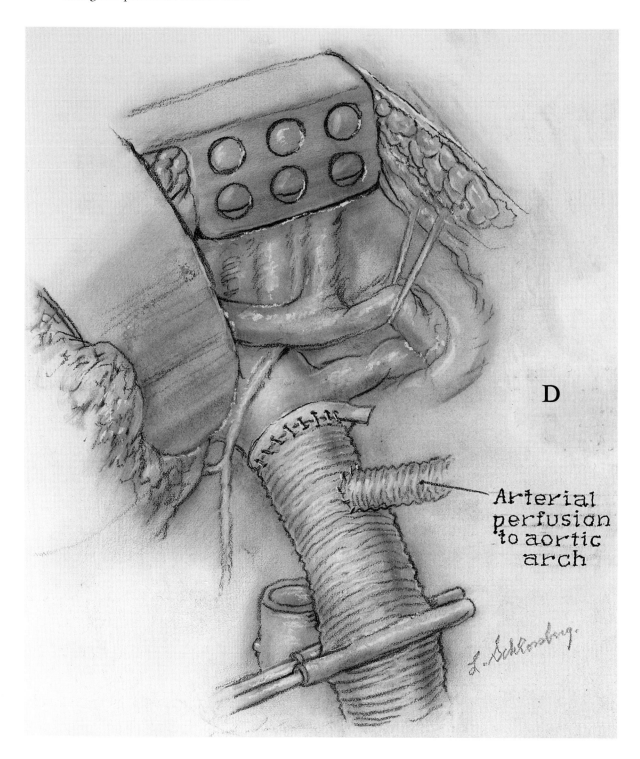

D

Arterial perfusion to aortic arch

E In preparation for the distal anastomosis, the descending thoracic aorta is transected. Teflon felt is used to reinforce the native tissue for the end-to-end anastomosis, performed with a running 3-0 monofilament nonabsorbable suture. Before completion of the anastomosis, the aorta and graft are de-aired by partial release of the distal and proximal clamps in sequence. Both clamps are then removed and perfusion continued through the 8-mm side-arm graft while the cannula to the left femoral artery side arm is clamped. The latter graft is transected close to the left femoral artery and oversewn. Rewarming is continued, and, once the nasopharyngeal temperature reaches 28° to 30° C, lidocaine is administered and the heart is defibrillated back to sinus rhythm.

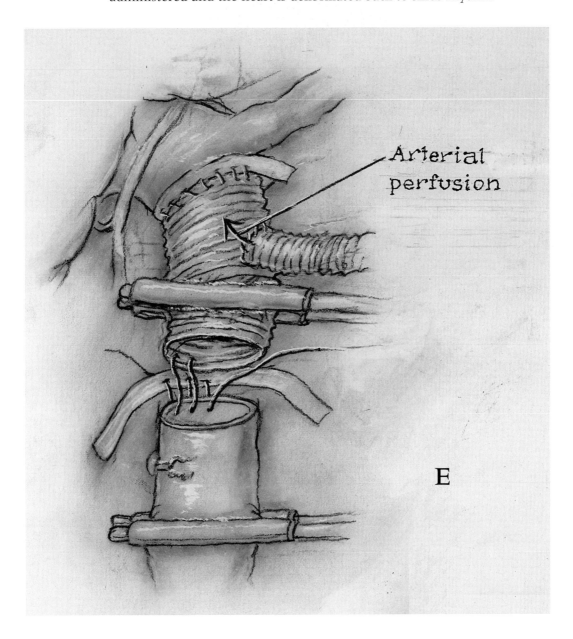

Arterial perfusion

E

F Once rewarming is complete and hemostasis of both proximal and distal suture lines confirmed, the heart is allowed to fill and eject, and the patient is separated from cardiopulmonary bypass. The left atrial cannula is removed and the purse-string tied and reinforced with 4-0 monofilament figure-of-eight suture. The cannula in the left femoral vein is removed and the purse-string suture at the saphenofemoral junction secured. The proximal stump of saphenous vein is oversewn. Next, the 8-mm side arm on the tube graft is ligated and divided if this graft was not used for an end-to-end anastomosis to the left subclavian artery. The remnant of the aortic wall may be sutured over the Hemashield graft. Once protamine is administered and hemostasis achieved at all cannulation sites and suture lines, the incisions are closed in standard fashion with two chest tubes placed anteriorly and posteriorly in the left pleural space.

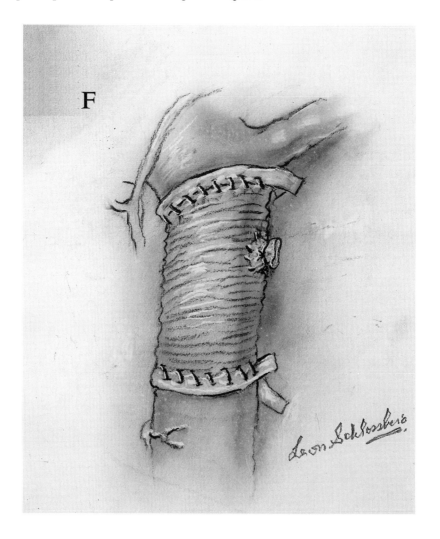

Chapter 24

Repair of Thoraco-abdominal Aneurysms Involving the Distal Aortic Arch

G. Melville Williams, M.D.

Fusiform or Degenerative Aneurysms

It is rare that a degenerative aneurysm of the descending thoracic aorta will extend to the distal aortic arch. More commonly, the entire ascending aorta, arch, and proximal descending aorta are involved in the degenerative process. Surgical repairs should begin proximally, replacing the ascending aorta and arch through a median sternotomy. There is generally some rim of tissue at the origin of the left subclavian artery facilitating an anastomosis so that the elephant trunk procedure can be performed if necessary. This allows the second stage to proceed in a much simpler fashion, obviating the need for cold circulatory arrest which would otherwise be necessary. When the distal arch is involved, cold circulatory arrest is required in most cases to achieve sufficient exposure for a safe anastomosis.

Acute Aortic Dissection

Aortic dissections originating in the distal arch are treated best as true proximal tears requiring emergency surgery via median sternotomy. In fact, we have come to the realization that tears starting inferior to the left subclavian artery which extend proximally despite medical management should always undergo emergency repair.

A-B Dissections beginning distinctly inferior to the origin of the left subclavian artery require repair for rupture or expansion, manifest by continued or recurrent symptoms or by CT or transesophageal echocardiography evidence of increased diameter. We believe that dissections occurring in a relatively normal-sized aorta and beginning distal to the left subclavian artery and resulting in branch occlusion are best treated by distal (meaning abdominal) catheter fenestration or surgical membranectomy.

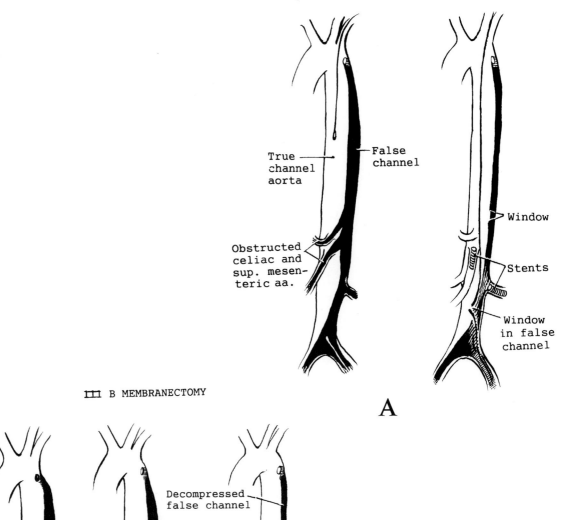

True
channel
aorta

False
channel

Obstructed
celiac and
sup. mesen-
teric aa.

Window

Stents

Window
in false
channel

A

⊞ B MEMBRANECTOMY

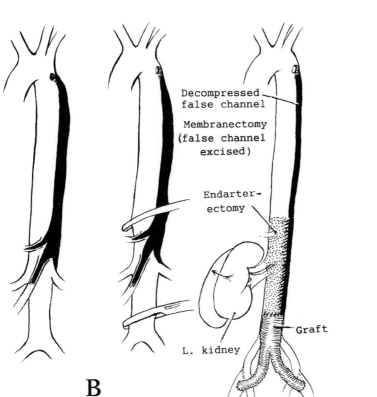

Decompressed
false channel

Membranectomy
(false channel
excised)

Endarter-
ectomy

Graft

L. kidney

B

Artwork in this chapter originally appeared in Stone CD, Williams GM: Ann Thorac Surg 57:580–587, 1994.

Chronic Dissection

Dilatation of the proximal descending thoracic aorta is the most common late complication of a chronic aortic dissection. In most instances, the aorta is sound at or just inferior to the take-off of the left subclavian artery, while in others the aneurysm may well balloon out, displacing the left subclavian artery medially, making it unwise to try to dissect the aorta distal to the left subclavian artery for the purpose of clamping. Patients presenting with this type of anatomy are best evaluated by three-dimensional CT scans employing contrast. The precise anatomic relationships of the arch branches to the aneurysm can be determined and decisions can be made regarding the need for cold circulatory arrest.

Surgical Exposure

The availability of superb and versatile retractors fixed to the operating room table have proved invaluable. Prior to their application, we commonly chose to make a long thoraco-abdominal skin incision and to do a double thoracotomy, resecting the fifth rib for proximal exposure and the ninth interspace to conclude the repairs of the thoracic aorta. With the new retractors, equivalent exposure can be achieved by excision of the sixth rib, division of the costal margin, and removing a segment of the fifth rib posteriorly. The retractors can open this incision sufficiently well to replace the entire descending thoracic and abdominal aorta in most patients.

In most patients requiring repair of the distal aortic arch, the phrenic and vagus nerves may be freed with overlying pleura from the aorta. While we try in all cases to preserve the vagus nerve and its recurrent laryngeal branch, our patients are informed of the likelihood for a subsequent operation to medialize the left vocal cord. These procedures are so successful that we are less concerned with nerve preservation than previously.

The Management of Cold Circulatory Arrest

The left femoral artery and vein are exposed. An 8-mm woven graft or collagen-impregnated woven graft is anastomosed end-to-side to the left common femoral artery for inflow. We prefer this rather than directly cannulating the femoral artery, which renders the left leg ischemic for the period of time required for repair. The heartport venous catheter is inserted through the saphenous vein right at the sapheno-femoral junction over a guide wire into the right atrium. Its position is confirmed by transesophageal echocardiography. The left inferior pulmonary vein is then cannulated with a right-angle drainage catheter for decompression of the left ventricle. This set-up has allowed for very satisfactory cardiopulmonary bypass.

C   Alternatively, the pulmonary artery may be cannulated for venous return as shown. The distal arch should be dissected sufficiently to identify the left subclavian and left carotid arteries. However, in many instances, particularly in patients who have had a prior repair of the ascending aorta, scar tissue in the proximity of the great vessels prevents full exposure, which is deferred until circulatory arrest. The site for the distal anastomosis is now prepared and the aorta controlled at this point.

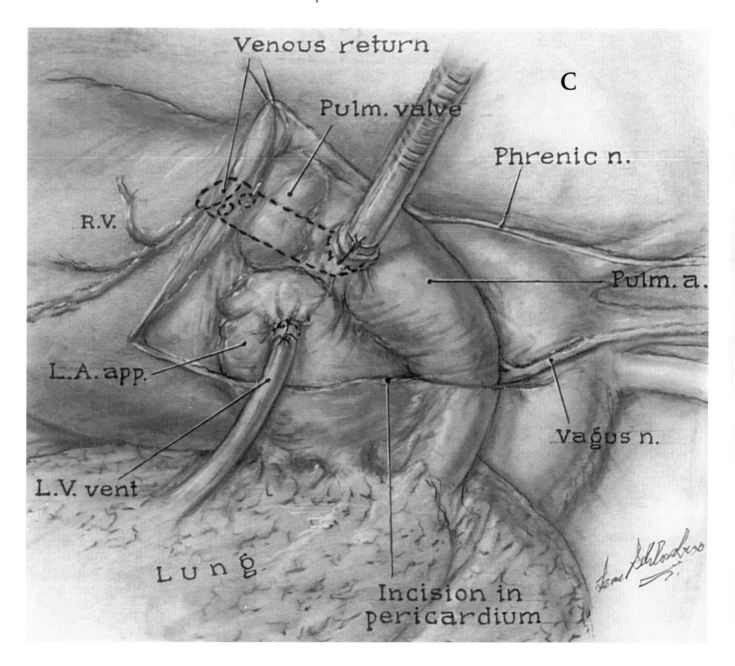

Aneurysm Repair

We advocate lowering body temperature to 32°C for partial left heart bypass and 18° C for circulatory arrest. During the period of cooling, which is tedious, attempts should be made to identify and ligate every intercostal and bronchial artery deemed unimportant as a source of blood supply to the spinal cord. This decision is made in large part by preoperative assessment of the spinal cord blood supply by selective injections of the intercostal arteries. Clipping these vessels to control backbleeding before the aneurysm is opened greatly reduces blood loss and reduces ischemic time. When circulatory arrest is employed, an 8-mm woven hemishield graft is sutured to the side of the woven graft chosen for replacing the aneurysm. This "branch" provides a means for reintroducing circulation to the heart and head as soon as the proximal aortic anastomosis is completed, thereby reducing the time of circulatory arrest in this predominantly elderly population.

When the bladder temperature has reached 18° C and after 30–45 minutes of cooling, the aorta is clamped in the mid-descending thoracic aorta. Slow-flow perfusion is sustained to the viscera and the legs, while the blood volume from the upper half of the body is drained into the reservoir.

D   The aorta is opened proximally. In the case of aortic dissection, the extent of the membrane is clearly identified by opening into both channels. The aorta is then completely transected so that it is absolutely clear that anastomotic sutures are passing through the entire aortic wall, including adventitia. Most often, this leaves an oblique opening at the arch with the inferior portion more proximal than the superior portion, which includes the left subclavian artery. The graft is cut obliquely to match this opening. A strip of teflon felt 1-cm wide is attached to the transected proximal aorta with 4 or 5 mattress sutures, a step which simplifies the proximal anastomosis and keeps the felt on the aortic side. We have not used an inner layer of teflon felt unless the dissection extends into the anterior arch. If so, the false channel is obliterated.

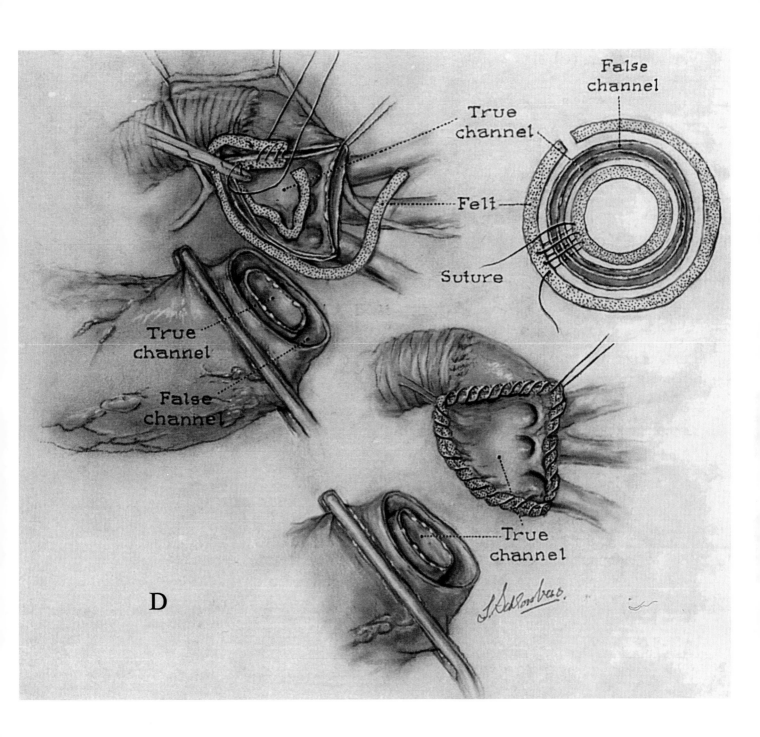

False
channel

True
channel

Felt

Suture

True
channel

False
channel

True
channel

D

Aneurysm Repair *continued*

E   Simple coapting suture technique is used and, after completion of the anastomosis, volume is restored and de-airing is carried out through the graft itself. The limb which had been sutured to the graft (see Figure I) is now cannulated, and split perfusion and rewarming are begun.

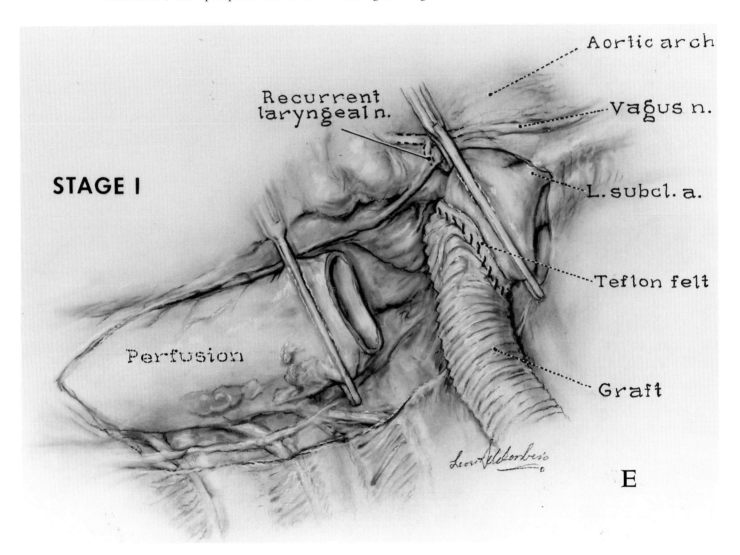

F-H When the descending thoracic and abdominal aorta are greater than 4 cm in diameter, the intercostal and visceral arteries are implanted sequentially.

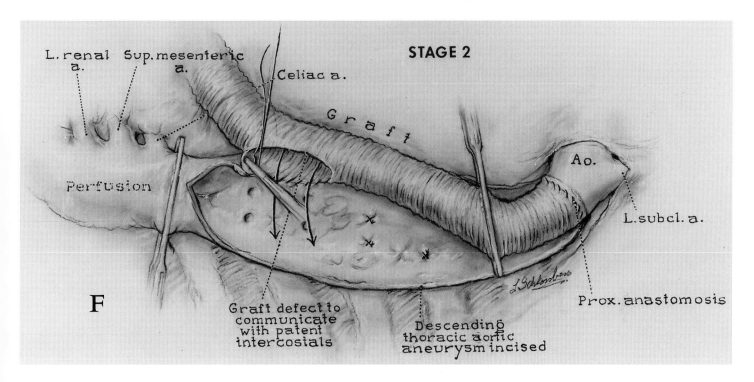

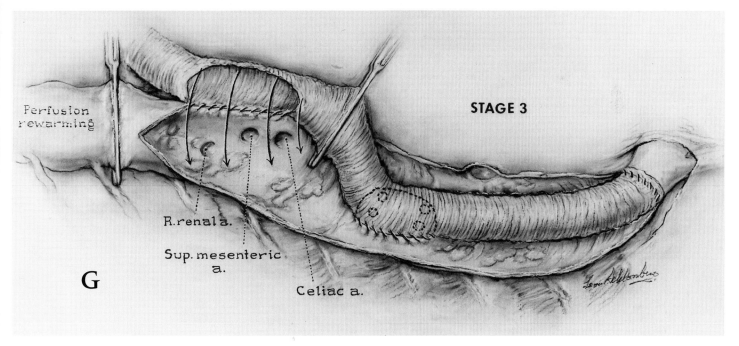

Aneurysm Repair *continued*

F-H *continued*

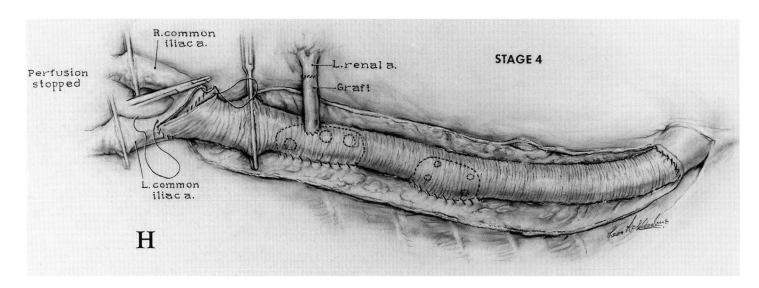

H

I-K In cases of aortic dissection where the aorta is not aneurysmal from the mid-chest inferiorly, the membrane is resected.

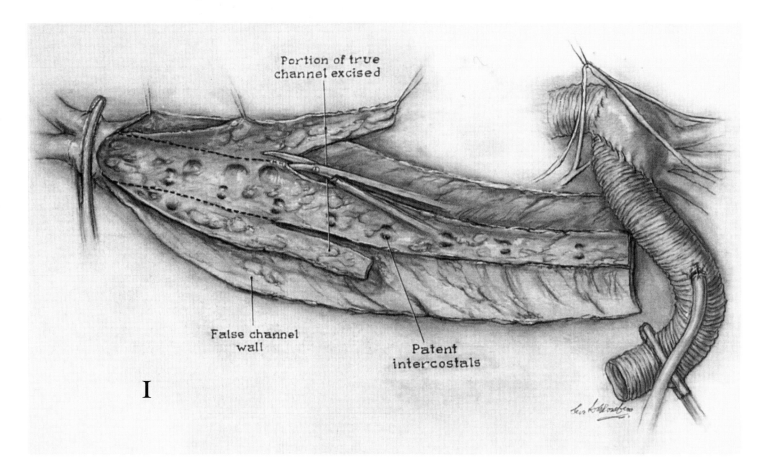

I

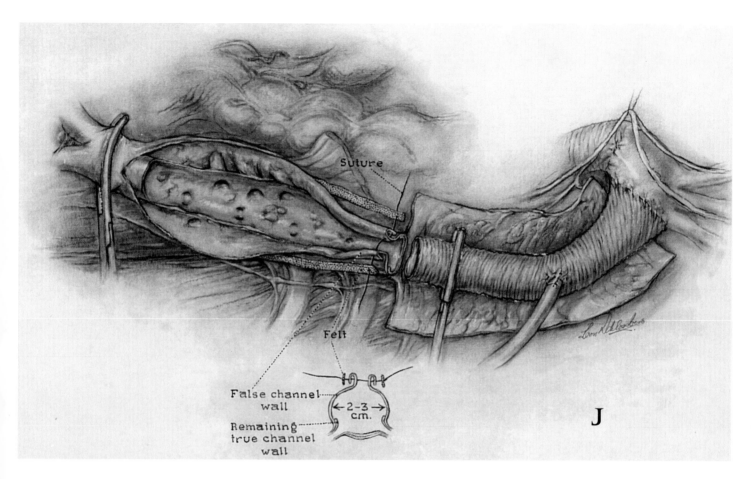

Suture

Felt

False channel
wall

Remaining
true channel
wall

2-3
cm.

J

K

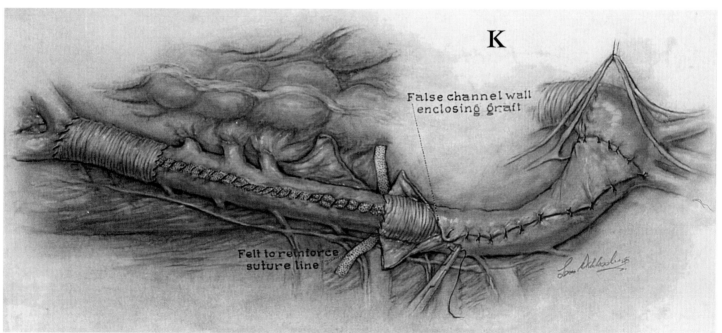

False channel wall
enclosing graft

Felt to reinforce
suture line

The period of rewarming may be extremely tedious as it is commonly associated with oozing, which is only partly remedied by closure of the aneurysm sac over the graft. The surgeon must be compulsive in obtaining hemostasis.

Chapter 25

Repair of Fusiform Aneurysms of the Descending Thoracic Aorta

G. Melville Williams, M.D.

Introduction

With the advent of better and better techniques for the introduction and placement of stent grafts, open surgery for the repair of fusiform aneurysms of the descending thoracic aorta is likely to be reserved for the most extensive and complicated cases. Thus, while surgery for the repair of a mid-descending thoracic aorta localized fusiform aneurysms is simple and straightforward, patients will choose the stent graft, as recovery from femoral artery cutdown is far easier than from a thoracotomy. Special circumstances requiring thoracotomy include (1) close proximity to the aortic arch and/or celiac axis, (2) advanced atherosclerosis of the iliac vessels, and (3) aneurysm involving the entire descending thoracic aorta and proximal abdominal aorta. The management of aneurysms involving the distal arch is described in the previous chapter.

The Role for Partial Left Heart Bypass

Controversy still remains about the value of partial left heart bypass, which involves a groin incision and the potential risk of infection. Cannulating the left side of the heart also adds the risk of introducing air. We find these potential problems outweighed by the advantage of performing deliberate and careful anastomoses. Further, the heart is easily unloaded, which we find important in elderly patients, half of whom have had or continue to have significant coronary artery disease.

Operative Management

A   The patient is positioned as for a standard left posterolateral thoracotomy. The eighth or ninth interspace is selected for aneurysms involving the lower half of the descending thoracic aorta, and the sixth rib is resected and the costal margin divided in instances in which the entire descending thoracic aorta must be replaced. Alternatively, a double thoracotomy provides the best exposure for stout patients. A standard posterolateral thoracotomy skin incision is made and the chest entered by resection of the fifth rib and incising the ninth interspace without division of the costal margin. The diaphragm does not need to be divided, for the superior portion of the abdominal aorta can be visualized and controlled easily by enlarging the aortic hiatus at the diaphragm.

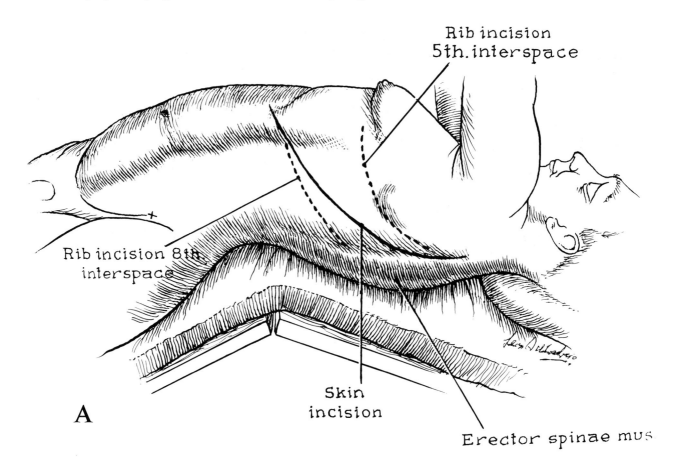

While one team is doing the thoracotomy, a second exposes the left femoral vessels. In the obese patient, the incision is best made obliquely above the groin crease to keep the incision away from the macerated groin area. The common femoral artery immediately inferior to the inguinal ligament is dissected easily.

Artwork in this chapter originally appeared in Williams GM, Schlossberg L: Atlas of Aortic Surgery. Baltimore, Lippincott-Williams & Wilkins, 1997.

B In general, the surgical dissection for the control of the descending thoracic aorta is very straightforward. The plane adjacent to the normal aorta is easily identified. In some patients, large veins are present posterior to the descending thoracic aorta, and in all cases the thoracic duct is not far away. By staying right next to the aorta, these structures can be avoided. To gain control just inferior to the subclavian artery, sharp dissection to divide the ligamentum arteriosum is necessary. Once this structure is cut, control of the aorta is easy to establish.

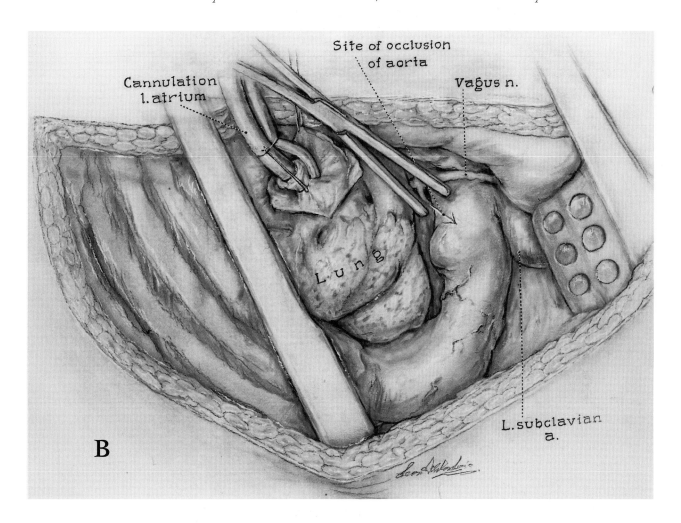

Once the aortic and femoral dissections have been completed, the patient is heparinized, providing a hundred units/kg body weight. The atrium or the left inferior pulmonary vein is now identified and dissected. A purse-string suture of 2-0 Tevdek is placed and a plastic right angle drainage catheter is introduced through a stab wound made with an 11 blade as the anesthesia team provides positive pressure. As the catheter is introduced, the purse string is tightened using a Rumel tourniquet. The catheter is tied to the red rubber tubing of the Rumel with heavy braided silk. Simultaneously, the surgical assistant attaches an 8-mm woven collagen-impregnated graft end-to-end to the common femoral artery. This graft is now cannulated with a size 22 or 24 catheter. The left heart and common femoral artery catheters are now connected via the centrifugal pump. A small catheter is introduced over a guide wire in the femoral artery graft to monitor distal pressure. Partial bypass is now begun.

Operative Management *continued*

C The proximal anastomosis is begun employing the "parachute" technique. The most difficult area of the anastomosis from the point of view of exposure is addressed first, and this is usually the right inferolateral portion of the aorta as illustrated; 3-0 polypropylene sutures have performed very satisfactorily in our experience. The use of a teflon felt buttress makes the anastomosis somewhat more cumbersome, but prevents needle-hole bleeding in most cases and, as a result, saves time. As shown, the distal clamp on the descending thoracic aorta is placed immediately adjacent to the divided aorta, obviating backbleeding from the bronchial or intercostal arteries while allowing perfusion of these vessels through the pump.

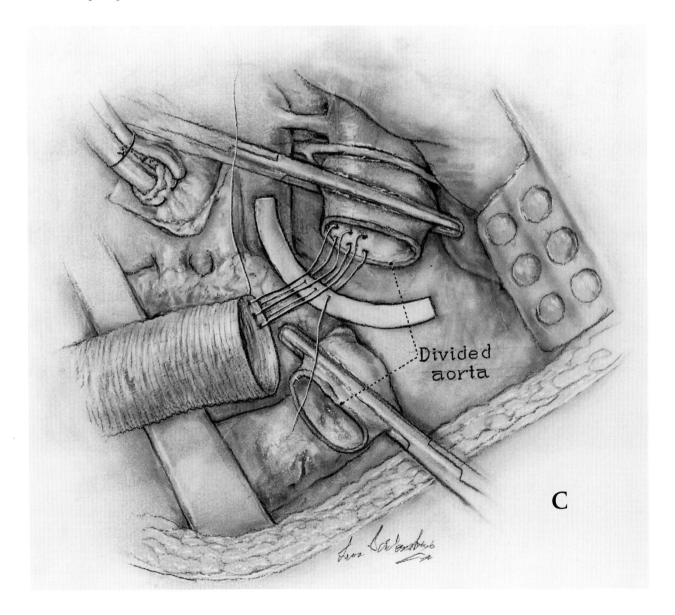

D The aortic clamp is then moved distally beyond the aneurysm. Recently, with the aneurysm decompressed, we have found it simple to dissect and clip the intercostal arteries judged not to be important for spinal cord perfusion, usually those in the upper two thirds of the descending thoracic aorta. This maneuver greatly reduces backbleeding and the time spent oversewing these vessels when the aneurysm is opened.

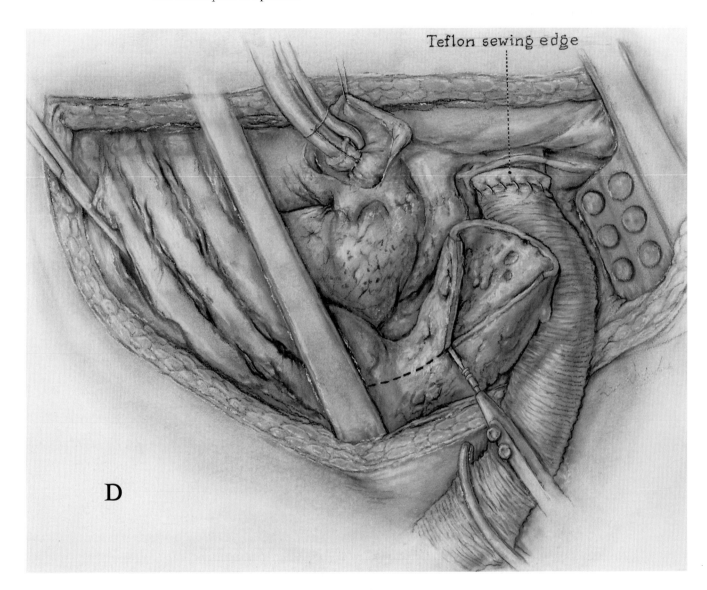

D

Operative Management *continued*

E   The aneurysm is opened laterally using the cautery, and residual backbleeding vessels are oversewn with figure-eight sutures of 3-0 prolene.

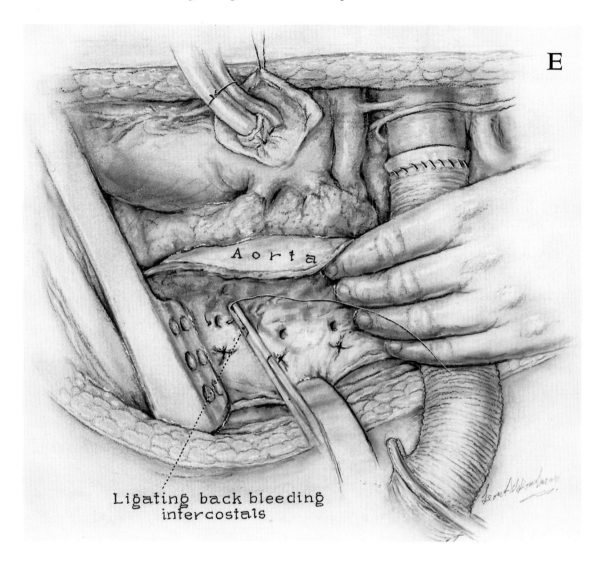

Ligating back bleeding intercostals

F   The distal anastomosis is completed.

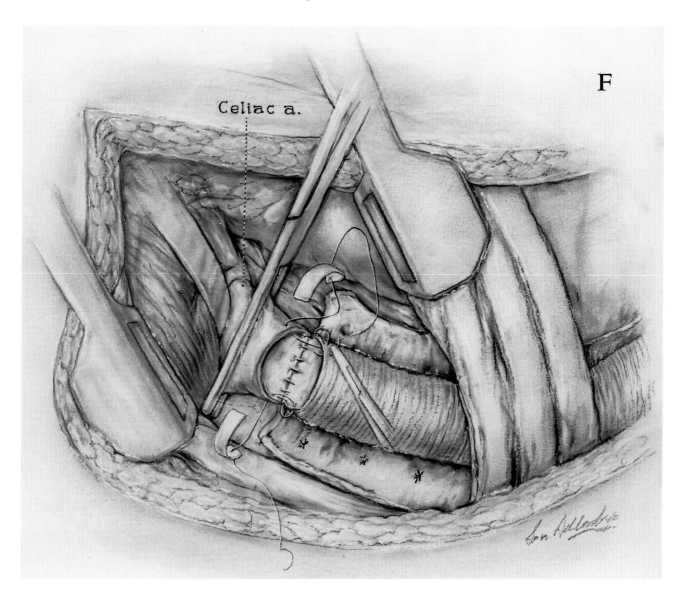

Operative Management *continued*

G The aneurysm sac or pleura is closed about the graft, shielding it from possible pleural space contamination.

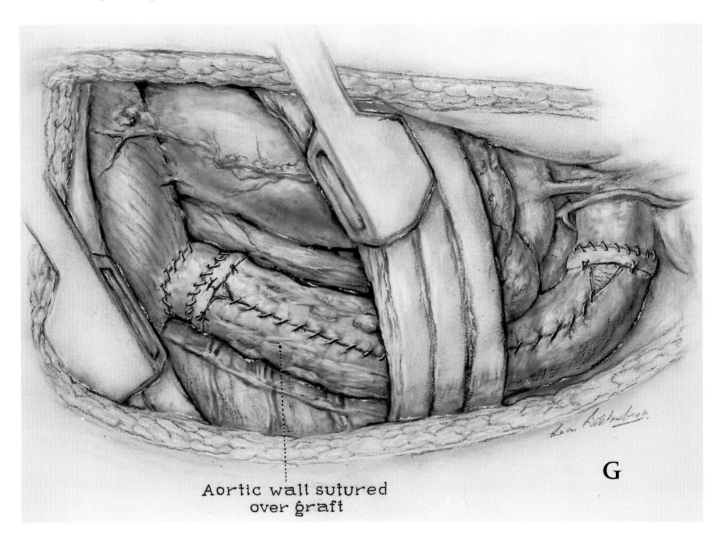

Aortic wall sutured over graft

G

The Prevention of Paraplegia

The great radicular artery (artery of Adamkiewicz) arises as a branch of an intercostal artery anywhere from T-6 to L-2. It varies not only in location but also in size. The replacement of short segments of descending thoracic aorta seldom leads to paraplegia largely because there is a rich anastomotic network between the intercostal arteries such that the sacrifice of two to three pairs seldom causes spinal cord ischemia. This is why paraplegia is so rare after the deployment of stent grafts. Concern arises when the entire descending thoracic aorta must be repaired. Under these circumstances, we try diligently to preoperatively identify the source of the great radicular artery by selective injections of the intercostal vessel. In addition to identifying the source of the great radicular artery, this form of angiography also confirms the presence or absence of collaterals between the intercostal branches. Consequently, if the great radicular artery arises from T-10 but the aneurysm extends to below T-11, we would plan to incorporate the intercostal pair at T-11 in the distal anastomosis while sacrificing the pair at T-10 if we knew there were adequate collaterals between these branches. Spinal fluid drainage is also part of our protocol to reduce the incidence of paraplegia as much as possible.

Index